AMERICAN
BIOHACKER

RUSS SCALA

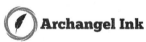

CONTENTS

PREFACE

I've observed a wide range of human behavior: murder, incest, infidelity, child abuse, drug addiction, spousal abuse, suicide, corruption. I've looked into patients' eyes and held their hands as I told them everything would be ok, when I knew they were going to die in minutes. I've hugged mothers on emergency scenes whose children were killed. I've been covered in every type of body fluid, including brain matter.

I've witnessed the heart of darkness, the unexplainable, and people who've shown generosity, compassion, and integrity that just blew my hair back. I've acquired a unique skill set from over 40 years in medicine and learned how to navigate the broken medical system to get people answers at the eleventh hour. This is my story.

Russ Scala

Winter Park, Florida

DEDICATION

I am writing this book as a form of therapy after finding both my mother and father dead inside their home just a few months ago. My DNA is hardwired with all that they taught me. I have modeled their behavior throughout my life. It has protected me in many dangerous situations and helped me understand people at their core. As a high-level interventionist, I use the skills they taught me every hour of every day when I meet new clients and get them the help they need. I know both my parents would be proud.

I love and miss you, Mom and Dad.

I still can't believe you're gone.

INTRODUCTION

As I write these lines, I'm in a dark place. The voices, memories, and sounds in my head are lighting up like fireworks during Chinese New Year. I can't shut my brain off. I've only felt this way once before, and I learned that the only way around it is to go straight through, so let's dive right in and get this party started.

After spending years responding to emergency calls as a paramedic and being attached to a SWAT team, not much worried or scared me, but that was all about to change as I flipped on the morning news.

An alert sounded and my picture flashed across the TV screen. A multi-agency criminal task force was raiding my company and the report was going live. The building was locked down and four people in management were being cuffed and taken away, charged with distributing performance-enhancing drugs.

My heart began to race… four had been arrested, and as Director of Research and Development, I knew I was next. At any second, the front door to my home was going to fly off the hinges, followed by agents throwing me to the floor. My mind was moving a million miles a minute. I could not focus and my thoughts were fueled by adrenaline. *How had this happened?* All my research on heart disease and diabetes, the testing I'd done on athletes… all of it would be forever tainted by this arrest. *Was I going to jail? Should I call someone?*

Stepping out of my panic for a moment, I looked at the TV again, and my picture was now on the screen with Dr. Claire Godfrey, one of the physicians that had been arrested. I had done a magazine cover with her a few months back and the media was using that picture of us to lead the story. Flipping between channels, I saw that the magazine cover was being used across all the networks. The news anchor was prattling on, "Next up, the names of the professional athletes and celebrities that used performance-enhancing drugs."

That's impossible! How had they gotten patients' names? I felt the urge to run. I certainly didn't want to stay at the house. I had worked on a SWAT team and knew what a dynamic entry was. I didn't want to be around for that. I jumped inside my black Porsche and drove downtown. My cell phone started ringing madly five minutes later. *How was I going to put all these fires out?* My brain was dropping screens and algorithms—I was hoping they'd show me what to do next.

Actually, let me stop here, while I have your attention, and tell you how all this started. This will be good for me… and anyone reading these lines may learn a thing or two.

Chapter One

SO IT BEGINS...

Now that I'm sliding into 60 years of age, I can look back and reflect on the chain of events that led me to develop eleventh-hour interventions for people. The fact is, life has kicked my ass and cursed me with the memories of many people dying in my arms. But I had exceptional parents who gave me the street smarts to question everything yet still somehow find the good in people. They made sure I was aware that priests, cops, teachers, doctors, politicians, Little League coaches, and everyone else, for that matter, were all capable of very bad things. Nothing is as it seems. Always do what you love and it will never seem like work. They were big on lessons like that. I love my mom and dad and miss them both.

My initial fascination with the human body started when I was eight years old. I was riding in the front seat with my father on Avenue A, in Bayonne, New Jersey. A strange sound rang out, like someone had kicked an empty box, as a guy on a bicycle was cracked by a car and ejected right in front of us. I remember the sudden jerk forward as my father braked to a quick stop. We both got out and a crowd immediately formed around the unconscious man. I saw fear growing in the eyes of the gathering crowd. No one was reacting. The victim's body was bent into a distorted position and blood streamed from his ears and eyes. An expanding urine stain darkened the man's gray pants. I remember not being afraid, just in a state of wonderment. My father opened the man's mouth and turned his head to the side, allowing the blood to drain. The blood had been blocking his airway, and we soon heard the hiss of air leaving his lungs. Dad was the only person there to take any action. When the ambulance arrived, my father and I got back in the car. He looked at me and said, "Ya good?"

I said, "Yes," and we got on with the day, as if nothing had happened. My father had reacted to and handled a situation that would paralyze most people. Did this start me on my way to becoming what I am today? Who knows… but I remember wanting to know why the blood coming from the man's ears was a different color than that of the laceration on his thigh.

At around fourteen, I went to work at the Bayonne Hospital to save lives, but I ended up lugging food trays to the rooms of sick people. Not the best job in the world, but I felt like I was in a museum, exploring every part of the hospital alphabet—CCU, ICU, ER— and listening and talking to people who were sick. It made me feel important. Most patients had no one to talk to.

It wasn't until our family moved to Florida that I got more involved with real hospital action. My father's brother, Dr. Raymond Scala, opened the doors for me at the Winter Park Emergency Department. He had founded Harbor School for special-needs children and had shared an intense interest in medicine with my father. They were both visionaries, to say the least.

While working as a union president, my father was called in many times to deal with workers who had mental issues or were struggling with alcoholism. He would take these people into our home and facilitate interventions. As a kid, I didn't understand his skill set, and my father was intense and to the point, which didn't always help. One time I came home from school to find a man staring at the wall of our day room. When I asked my father what was wrong, he pointed to our new guest and tapped his head with his index finger. "You figure out what goes on in here and you can help people deal with all the bullshit out there," he finished, pointing out the window.

Winter Park High School was surreal. I had no idea that I had ADHD—or dyslexia, for that matter—but while in class, I felt like I was running through waist-high snow. I just moved way too slow. Ironically, I was obsessed with the fast pace and energy of the emergency room where two physicians, Dr. Wurtzel and Dr. Corvelli— my mentors—would split shifts, taking me with them from room to room and explaining complex physiological reactions to medication. They pointed out the signs and symptoms of congestive heart failure, distended neck view, shallow respiration from fluid buildup in the lungs, and so much more. This was a place where every minute counted to save lives. The emergencies included spinal injuries, gunshot wounds, delivery of babies, heart attacks, and other life-threatening situations. I felt exhilarating anticipation when a cardiac arrest patient was brought back to life.

My first drug—and drug of choice—was adrenaline. I was right in the mix of everything and it was intoxicating. My time in the ER felt like being part of a gang, and nothing else seemed to matter. For example, I didn't understand the importance of learning algebra in high school. *Honestly, what was the point?* But when studying dosage calculations to administer medications by the milligram in emergency situations... *Bang! I got it.* I started skipping school just to work in the

ER. I had two physicians who were not only my mentors, but were also really cool guys who saw potential in me that my teachers missed.

I remember Dr. Wurtzel pulling me aside and telling me, "Russ, when we can move this equipment from the ER into the streets, then we'll really save some lives." As though he had a crystal ball, that's exactly what happened.

A perfect storm created the new paramedic program. It involved research released by NASA, which used telemetry to monitor astronauts' heart rate in space, and the procedures developed by medics in Vietnam, who began using intravenous solutions to maintain blood pressure from gunshot wounds. The new paramedic program soon spread across the US. I was one of the first in line. *Let's do this!*

Paramedic school was a blur. I became proficient in intravenous therapy, intubation, defibrillator use, MAST suit use, advanced cardiac life support, and drug therapy. I absorbed everything in the book on EKGs and how to detect deadly heart arrhythmia, and memorized complex physiological processes, as well as what drugs either sped up or slowed down the heart.

Ironically, we were not taught how to take care of ourselves. Instead, we learned the behaviors and coping mechanisms that emergency service folks needed to get through every shift. A poor diet, drinking, and occasionally popping pills during a shift were all seen as normal because we were saving lives. Our own bodies became collateral damage.

No one talked about what would happen to *us* after years of responding to emergency calls. You might not be aware, but cops, firemen, and paramedics all have a nasty habit of dying early from heart disease. We thought we were young and bulletproof, but we were wrong.

Working in the emergency room with a group of highly trained specialists was a chaotic yet carefully controlled dance. I studied how every medication was given intravenously, along with the exact time interval and milligram dose. As a paramedic responding first in a shooting, a whole new skill set had to be developed. Your patients' lives depended on it.

From our graduating class, many of the recruits went to work for NASA, which meant great pay, sleeping all night, and responding to very few calls... cushy duty. Of course, that didn't work for me. I wanted to be in the action and make a difference, so I went down to South Orange Blossom Trail, a dangerous part of Orlando, like the South Side of Chicago today. I worked 48 hours straight, without sleep, responding day and night to the most horrendous scenes a person could imagine. One ambulance covered 523 square miles. High-speed auto accidents, shootings, drug dealers and strippers beating each other to a bloody pulp... and that was all before midnight. For me, the lights and sirens were electric and I loved it. Smoking on the way to calls relaxed me and made me hyperfocused so when I arrived, I could do what I'd been trained to do. Nicotine, which we now know is a nootropic, calms neurotransmitters while simultaneously helping with intense focus. That's why smoking on the way to an emergency scene dialed me in. In a strange twist of fate, my ADHD gave me a distinct advantage. It was a curse in the traditional school model but a gift while considering the multiple things that could go sideways at any emergency scene.

You always remember your first fuck-up. It's burned into your memory forever.

The alarm blared and the dispatcher barked, "Unit 51 respond to car versus tree on 456 Palmer Ave." I clicked the sirens on and our response time was six minutes. More than enough time to light up a Marlboro Red, drag deep, and let that nicotine shoot across my blood-brain barrier. In four minutes, I would be jacked into the scene, ready to go to work.

We arrived and determined there was no gas leak and no wires down on the vehicle. Most citizens miss this and get killed trying to help people. I ran up to the car and made a quick assessment: impact speed of about 60 MPH, no seatbelt, patient had multiple lacerations on both arms, and a compound fracture from holding the steering wheel during impact. I called ahead to the trauma center. We needed to load and go. The guy was bleeding internally and had about a minute before he bled out. I started two IVs of Ringer's lactate while my crew stabilized his C-spine and prepped for transport.

When we arrived at the ER, we moved the patient to trauma room one, where physicians and teams were waiting. As they rolled the patient to a table, X-rays were ordered, blood was taken, and my crew left the ER, returning to the rescue truck. As we were cleaning up, the attending ER physician walked out of the ER, approached me, and said, "Your patient was shot three times in the chest. How did you miss that?"

I stood there, dumbfounded. I was a rookie and had only seen a car versus tree, when in reality, the man had been shot three times, got in his car, passed out from blood loss, and hit the tree. This was one of my first calls as a paramedic, but the doctor was right... *How did I miss that?*

When you pull up to a scene, you're taught to make a quick evaluation. All I saw was a mangled car smashed into a tree; a shooting was the furthest thing from my mind. It had been a small caliber gun, and the bullet wounds were mixed with small lacerations. I had focused on the bones protruding from his arms and completely missed the bullet wounds. However, I can tell you one thing: nothing like that ever happened again.

Chapter Two

DEAD AIR

For about 200 years, medicine treated the head separately from the rest of the body, when in fact, brain chemistry is deeply interconnected with multiple metabolic systems. Back in the day, while off duty, we would drink. Cops, firemen, and paramedics all hung out together, along with a good supply of nurses and ER groupies. Early on in a stressful career, your brain chemistry takes the first hit. The excess cortisol caused by stress lowers the feel-good neurotransmitters: serotonin, dopamine, and adrenaline. When these neurotransmitters are low, there are different ways to elevate them. Carbohydrates, like bread, white rice, beer, or pasta (poor man's Prozac), as well as nicotine, caffeine, and opiates all work.

We medicated ourselves with alcohol, simple carbohydrates, and prescription drugs, keeping our serotonin levels elevated. We even called beer "liquid bread." Chronic stress leads to elevated cortisol levels, effectively shutting down protective hormonal responses. That includes your thyroid and adrenal hormones, testosterone, estrogen, and growth hormones. When all of those protective responses are diminished, your body becomes ground zero for heart disease, diabetes, cancer, and depression. But no one knew that back then. We were just doing our jobs.

Years later, I would write advanced treatment protocols for war vets, emergency service personnel, and celebrity clients who were not getting answers from conventional medicine. But in the late 70s and early 80s, I was just trying to understand my own brain chemistry. I simply could not deal with regular people; I would always prefer to be with my team at work. This behavior was not healthy, but it took me a while to understand why.

New research shows that many artists, actors, comedians, scientists, and visionaries were born with DRD4, a dopamine gene, which causes them to have low circulating dopamine levels. Dopamine is a neurotransmitter known as one of the happiness hormones. Even the ping of a cellular phone causes a little squirt of dopamine. Here's the rub. When working extremely intense scenes, the lights, adrenaline bursts, fast-paced atmosphere, smells, and intense visuals also become feel-good chemicals. The job itself is highly addicting, especially if you were born with low dopamine levels. People with low dopamine gravitate towards exciting lines of work, and yes, I have low dopamine levels, but I wouldn't discover that for a while.

While off duty, life didn't move fast enough for me. And it's not just me. Dead air is the time when many high-functioning people get into trouble with drugs, alcohol, sex… anything for that dopamine burst. I'd be at the bar drinking, knowing that behavior was killing me. Eventually, I would call in to work and take a shift. I would rather be jacked in, running emergency calls and constantly being challenged, than drinking and just "existing" like an ordinary citizen. Maybe it's because I was the first born in my family. I was always fine on my own. I didn't need to date and didn't want buddies around me 24/7. I did like connecting with people who I thought were wicked smart and well read, as opposed to firemen and cops in my group who were saying, "I'm waiting on my twenty-year retirement… only ten more to go."

When I heard that, my gut would shrivel. *Fucking shoot me,* I'd think. I would rather be dead than think like that. After enough people died in my arms, I recognized that life can be over in a nanosecond. My dad used to say, "Do what you love to do and don't live above your means." Why opt in to golden handcuffs where you have to work just to keep your head above water? *Fuck that. Thanks for the advice, Dad.* That was no way to live.

One day, a patient who had been stabbed multiple times bled out and died en route as we careened to the trauma center. As I washed the blood from the floor of our rescue truck, before going to eat dinner with my crew, my partner said, "Brother, you're cold as ice. Don't you ever blink?"

That phrase always stuck with me. I understood where his comment came from, but it wasn't that I didn't care. It's just that I had a particular skill set and saw every situation like a stopwatch had just been clicked. I had minutes and I did my best, but when I failed, I had to move on. If I thought about each patient as a person with a family, considered what job he had or whether he'd kissed his wife that morning, I would never be able to work again. I had to be emotionally bulletproof, which came across to my partner as uncaring.

In the years to come, reality would reveal itself. I simply couldn't handle what I was seeing. Alcohol got me through the tough spots. *Ya think I was gonna talk to a counselor?* No way, we were men. Funny, as you age, your thinking changes. I didn't realize that the serotonin burst I got from alcohol, or the mood boost I got from copious amounts of empty carbs, was slowly killing me… but more on that later.

The paramedic program began sending me new recruits to train. A select group of paramedics are given the responsibility of being preceptors, and they mentor, oversee, and evaluate new paramedics in the field. Once new recruits graduate from paramedic school, they're sent to the relatively calm environment of a hospital to master IV administration, intubation, and defibrillation. After they had done that, I would bring the new recruits to the emergency scenes on the streets and basically let them practice their advanced lifesaving procedures on live patients. They were all good kids and were passionate about saving lives, but starting intravenous therapy upside down in a vehicle with a gas spill can make you second-guess your chosen line of work. I could always pick out the men and women who would make it; they had the ability to compartmentalize the emergency scene, put it in the back of their heads, and learn from it. War vets who made it out of battle without PTSD have the same ability.

I would always tell 'em straight up, "Don't make this your career. Don't be a lifer. Look around at the officers who've been on the job ten or twenty years. Their health is gone, they're obese, dealing with diabetes, taking antidepressant medication, and divorced, but still wearing golden handcuffs."

Of course, you have to work to pay the bills. One saving grace of the job was shift work—24 hours on, 48 hours off. The human metabolism can handle stress in intervals, which helps to increase longevity on the job.

The book *Why Zebras Don't Get Ulcers* speaks to the fight-or-flight stress response. I'll save you from reading 400 pages and cut to the heart of it. Research in psychoneuroimmunology shows that physical, mental, and emotional stress weakens your immune system. The stress hormone, cortisol, when elevated, can damage multiple metabolic systems, as well as brain, heart, and muscle tissue.

Back in the early 80s, we didn't know any better. Cops, firemen, paramedics, war vets... they were always the first through the fucking door, but the last to be taken care of. Is there any wonder why heart disease is the highest in this group? Research shows that the testosterone-to-cortisol ratio is one part of the problem. When you're hit with chronic stress, the elevated cortisol levels send your hormones into the toilet. Forget libido and muscle; testosterone is needed to keep your arteries dilated so oxygen and nutrients can get to your brain and heart and put up a shield.

The young recruits I trained all wanted to help people and be part of a team, and I do believe that it's hardwired into our DNA to help each other. I taught them: "As you evolve through this career path, the people you are saving are also killing you. You don't see it at first, and you don't feel it. It happens slowly."

All of us have a little Pac Man in our brain who gobbles up all the circulating adrenaline when we're young. As we age and our stress levels increase, the Pac Man gets slower. We start to cycle obsessively through thoughts and scenarios. *What if I did this or gave this drug first?* It's endless self-critique.

I would listen to people scream while looking them in the eyes on the way to the hospital. Knowing they were going to die never affected me. I would hold their hand and watch the heart monitor until it flatlined. In the beginning, I was fine, but after a few years, I would ruminate and see their faces. Soon, I was getting tears in my eyes. This is how elevated cortisol sneaks up on you. I'm in charge of fifteen people with millions of dollars of equipment, and if they see weakness in me, I'm done.

While training the new paramedics, I would make it a point to say, "Guys, you have to be selfish. Take care of yourself on your off days. Pick a sport and find a positive group outside emergency personnel. Do that or you'll become sleep-deprived, sedentary, malnourished, overfed, and socially isolated. How can regular people relate to what you do and how can you relate to what's important in their lives?"

Over the years, I've worked with many addicts, and just as we judge obese people for having "no will power"—which is totally false—we also think of addicts as bad people, with no one but themselves to blame. That is simply not true. The drugs just allow them to feel normal—for a while, at least. Likewise, after working emergency scenes, you just want to feel normal. Calming down your brain chemistry from being hyperalert is an art. Many fall into addiction, which they can often hide for years.

Research shows that your immediate peer group can either save you or kill you. When your peer group is the same as your work group, you never have time to decompress. You keep talking about the same topic, recalling possible mistakes and pain points, which causes the brain to hardwire bad thoughts. The off-duty drinking and partying was just part of it, but it wasn't sustainable behavior.

I loved my job. Nothing felt better than hooking a person up to the cardiac monitor, pressing a button, and sending a picture of the EKG to the emergency room physicians. I could increase the heart rate in third-degree heart block with .5 mg of atropine. I could stop a ventricular arrhythmia, called PVCs, with 75 mg of lidocaine. I was damn good at my job, and seeing the direct outcome of my work—saving lives and making a difference—became an addiction. Ordinary activities drove me crazy. I couldn't even handle a trip to Bed Bath & Beyond with my girl. Strolling five feet behind her as she compared pastel bath towels made me sick. I ended up being alone because I couldn't deal with everyday interactions with other people.

I had free reign in the hospital, asking medical staff questions and talking to patients. It was amazing training for me. I often wondered why one stroke patient would leave the hospital faster than another. *Why do some patients heal faster than others?* I was extremely curious and a pain in the ass, and I knew it. Through all of that, in the back of my mind was the guy on the bicycle who had been hit by a car when I was a kid. Intense visuals can get burned into your brain.

In your twenties, you're bulletproof, but my health was deteriorating, and I started to notice the signs and symptoms early. My diet was extremely high in carbohydrates because I needed that serotonin burst. I was not sleeping. My brain chemistry was out of balance, but I was too young to understand the dangers of excess cortisol splashing off my hippocampus. While I was off work, I found it impossible to deal with dead air. During downtime, on many occasions, I would call the department and say, "Let me come in and work a shift." As soon as the lights and sirens were turned on, I was back—completely dialed in—and I loved that feeling. I also wanted to pay my house off so I was working 96-hour shifts. Trust me, you don't need drugs to hallucinate. They taught us how to save lives, but they didn't teach us how to save ourselves.

Looking back, I was in hyperdrive and the only way I could feel good was to hack my body with carbohydrates, alcohol, nicotine, and adrenaline. I knew that something was wrong, but I was *not* going to a counselor. I didn't want that on my record, as it was a red flag for weakness. I had to compartmentalize my emotions.

You don't need a Ph.D. in psychoneuroimmunology to know that physical, mental, and emotional stress damages multiple metabolic systems and lowers immune surveillance. It was clear that most of the emergency service personnel were obese and had some illness already. I knew that I eventually had to move on. The money was great, but I felt like I was put on Earth to do something else.

There is a community among emergency personnel, like with war vets, and like any community, it can keep you safe and healthy... or it can kill you. One of my good friends, Joe Deholczer, was an artist and was constantly hazed at the fire department for being gay. Joe ended up committing suicide with a .45 to the chest. Yeah, we were a brotherhood alright.

After Joe killed himself, another paramedic friend of mine, Louie Salado, was killed by a car, a fact I couldn't get out of my head. *There was time,* I thought. Since we saved lives, we were protected, right? Well, with my two close friends dead, and my hands starting to shake, I had nowhere to turn.

Chapter Three

TRAINING DAZE

It was 1979 when I first I heard about the Ironman race: a 2.4-mile ocean swim, 112-mile bike race, and 26.2-mile marathon all rolled into one ultra-endurance event. This would be a pivotal moment in my life. My buddy, Wink Hines, was a swimmer in high school and another paramedic with the department. He was the one who showed me the *Sports Illustrated* magazine story about the three-part race. I was instantly intrigued by the new sport. "Wow, man… we could be one of the first! But you and I have never even run a mile… "

All that would soon change. Wink was tragically killed in an auto accident a short time later when he drove headlong into a tree. He was sorely missed. Since we were life savers, many of us thought that we were immune to tragedy, so a wake-up call like that kept me frosty, on the edge, hyperalert.

I knew I had to change my behaviors. I had to get away from the energy vampires. I started running because it felt good. The first time I ever ran, I could only cover half a mile. I was in terrible shape. I was bent over, my hands on my knees, heaving like a racehorse, and in my mind, I had just taken a beating. However, I liked that feeling; I liked it a lot. The next week, I covered a mile, and then two, and so it went.

Shift work allowed me to train almost full time. Twenty-four hours on, 48 hours off… that was how I lived most of my life. I would get off work and run a 6-mile loop; it was cleansing. It allowed me to process the events of the night before with clarity. This was my time to wipe the chalkboard clean in my head and start over. Working on people who are injured, and who will die within minutes if you don't save them, is defeating, so you must develop the ability to forget. After every run, the combination of sweat, heat, endorphins, and that dopamine bump allowed me to package that visual trauma, wrap it up, put a nice bow around it, and bury it in the back of my mind.

Running gave me a calmness I'd never felt before. Many times, while running, my foot strikes would sync with my breathing. I would enter a fugue state, gliding down the road for a 60-minute run that would only feel like five minutes. Later, I would use this as a tool with heroin addicts, but back then it just felt right for me. When I was done, I did not want a cigarette, or alcohol… I just wanted to relax, sit down, and read.

Running was my savior and my antidepressant; my feel-good neurotransmitters were all elevated after running. To me, running was a drug—my drug. I didn't care about racing or competing; it was medicinal. I had to leave my peers behind—the police and firemen—as this group was killing me with unhealthy coping mechanisms. As you can imagine, it's lonely when you have to make changes. But, I always keep moving forward, never looking back, and if you can't keep up with me, see ya later.

I was tripping on my brain chemistry daily, so starting to do endurance training in the early 80s may not have been the smartest thing to do. However, it did save me from some very bad behaviors to which I was gravitating.

The athletes that helped me were an amazing group of folks. I met Don Ardell and Jerry Gergley, two ultra-fit PhDs in their fifties at the University of Central Florida. I was thinking, *Cool, I have two more mentors,* and my God, were these guys fast. Don was a national champion and could run a six-minute mile at 55 years old. Jerry taught Exercise Physiology, and I trained for hundreds of miles with him. We became close friends. Triathlons were a brand-new sport and, as luck would have it, my group was on the tip of the spear.

I had a deep love for this type of training. In racing, you had to understand your metabolism. It was not about who was the fastest or strongest; it was about who knew their metabolism the best. It was a chess match between your brain and your body. Being able to race for five hours made you the mental and physical master of your body and the complex layers of performance, which include maintaining muscle and brain glycogen and keeping your metabolism firing on all cylinders.

Since I did not have any physical gifts, I developed friendships with people who were faster. Soon, these folks became my roommates and we traveled around Florida to race. The speed and talent in Winter Park was just stunning. We were home to some of the fastest people in the country. Two of them—Patrick Davis and Cole Blair—lived with me and part of the year Kent Richardson would come up from Bermuda to train in Orlando. I was so slow that I could only do the warm-up with them. I had no ego; I was just glad to be training with people who were so gifted.

It was a new beginning for me. I was applying my training in physiology, which soon allowed me to hack my own biology and calibrate my speed and recovery. I read everything about performance, studied for hours, and hired a swim coach to learn how to swim in open water, which was much different than training in a 25-meter pool. At the time, we were all looking for the best nutritional supplements to speed recovery from all those hours of training.

I would often do long training rides with a group that was in much better shape, which helped me reach the next level. I would hang out in the back of the cycling pack and do something called drafting, where you ride close behind another rider, allowing you to cut your expended effort in half. I would arrive at the 50-mile mark and could barely turn the pedals of the bike in a circle. I was so depleted that it was an effort just to get off the bike and walk into the store to buy fluids. My jet fuel was Coke; I would drink half of a 12oz can and within minutes I was back on the bike. I was riding like a god with no fatigue at all; that small amount of sugar and caffeine lit me up like a Christmas tree. Flat, de-fizzed Coke got me to quite a few finish lines.

Meanwhile, I was rooted in two cultures where I was able to glean insights and complete research to satisfy my continuous curiosity: emergency workers, who had the mental stress of responding to emergency calls, and endurance athletes, who had the physical stress of endurance training. Both groups of people were eating at least six meals per day, three main meals and two to three snacks. The simple carbohydrates increased serotonin levels and elevated insulin levels, which kept everyone hungry. I started researching why so many endurance athletes were putting on excess body fat, despite training for hundreds of miles.

Carbohydrates were king in 1984; that all changed for me in 1996 when I reviewed the research on mitochondria, which are the cellular factories that create energy. This research indicated that mitochondria burn fat better than carbohydrates for fuel, so we implemented the high-fat, low-carb diet, which was totally unheard of at that time. (Recently, Patrick Davis told the story on the Russ Scala YouTube channel.) Everyone thought we were crazy, but by that point, I didn't care what people thought. I trained for and completed the Victor 12.6-mile open water swim around Key West using that kind of high-fat diet. I knew that this would go mainstream. I expected every endurance athlete to soon be using this diet, but that didn't actually happen until 2015.

Over time, I realized the endurance racing was damaging my body, just like the stress of responding to rescue calls. At the time, I thought fast race times meant that I was healthy. I was so wrong, and one of the first signs I had was a dangerous cardiac arrhythmia called an atrial fib, when the top chamber of the heart, the atria, is beating so fast that the blood is never pushed out and can begin to clot. This situation scared the hell out of me. I went to four cardiologists, but got no answers. This was the beginning of my research into why endurance athletes so often need bypass surgery and stents. Racing at these levels damages the lining of the coronary arteries, called the endothelial lining. Many triathletes, including close friends of mine, have died from this endo-thelial dysfunction. It would take me fifteen years to prove what I already knew, but as I always say, "Roll with it, adapt, change, have fun… we're only here for a short period of time."

Working as a paramedic in my early twenties taught me that tomorrow may not happen, so live in the moment. With my under-standing of physiology, I knew that the elevated level of cortisol in my body was causing muscle wasting. This is called gluconeogenesis, where elevated cortisol from training rips into the muscle, first converting it to amino acids, then blood glucose. I always felt extremely bad—both physically and mentally—after long races. I would tear up at movies. I was unable to get an erection for months after a race. If I was so healthy, why did I feel this way? I knew this training was causing damage, but I justified it in my mind. I was not drinking, so this was the path I needed to be on… for the time being.

My race was the Half-Iron Man, Panama City, Florida. Flat, fast, and hot, I competed in a 1.5-mile swim, 56-mile bike ride, and 13-mile run. It took me 10 years to reach my peak in the sport. My first race took me 7 hours and 35 minutes; my last race 10 years later beat me down. I was on a 4-hour and 40-minute pace, but I blew up on the run, walked the last mile and a half, and finished in 5 hours and 5 minutes. I walked away from the sport, never to race again. I left it all out there on the course. I pushed my body and brain to places most people could never imagine. Later, I discovered that I had depleted almost all of my feel-good neurotransmitters, which explained why depression often followed races of that distance.

This was a sport that saved my life, but almost killed me at the same time. I had no idea that all the training was damaging my body, but I learned so much. It was the basis for the work I do helping endurance athletes today.

Chapter Four

THE POLICE ACADEMY & SWAT TEAM

My life was in overdrive and I had a big bull's-eye on my back. Firefighters may call themselves a brotherhood but, come promotion time, there is a lot of backstabbing and petty maneuvering. Brotherhood, my ass… like any other business, it was cutthroat.

The fire service represented 200 years of tradition, unaffected by progress. With the advanced technology in fire protection, there were a lot fewer fires, so fire departments had to justify their existence to mayors and city managers. This is where the paramedic system saved the fire service. With all the advanced lifesaving equipment paramedics had available, the emergency room could basically be moved into the streets, and manpower was needed to save lives. There were no more fires (not many at least), but there were a hell of a lot of emergency calls. For the record, the paramedic was in charge of the emergency scene, not the fire captain, who had been on the job for twenty years. The paramedics made more money, and the animosity was palpable.

Somehow, paramedics made a living saving lives, but it was a competitive sport. Every month, they would give out awards for communication on the emergency scene, and I was at the top of the list.

Raymond Beary, a boss-hog police chief, called me over one day after an emergency scene where I had shocked a heart attack victim back to life. He asked me if I would be willing to attend the police academy and be transferred to the SWAT team. I immediately said yes, so the right strings were pulled and, within a few months, I was a new recruit in the police academy.

The police academy had an interesting culture. There are three types of people who want to become cops: those who truly want to help people, those who need a job, and those who are bat-shit crazy. It did not take long to spot that last group. It's like panning for gold in every conversation; you get nuggets of information that quickly let you know that this guy is going to hurt people and is in the job for all the wrong reasons.

I was the first paramedic placed on the SWAT team in Winter Park. *Why? Did I know someone? Was it a political favor? Was it because I was a good guy?* It was because, whether you liked me or not, every police officer that watched me work said, "I want that guy working on me if I get shot." The bull's-eye on my back was now the size of a dinner plate. Cops and firemen were both trying to sabotage my efforts because they thought the mayor and city manager were going to combine police and fire into one group to save money. I was the test to see if it could be done, so a few administrators tried to make my life miserable. I just said, "Bring it." It's this political bullshit that slows down innovation. I had to go to the city commission three times to get approval for hepatitis shots for my crew. As always, the first people through the door are the last ones to be taken care of.

My job on the SWAT team was to stay behind with the snipers if an officer in the tactic team took a bullet. I would then move into the hot zone to start advanced life support, like a war medic, while contacting the trauma center to get the surgery room ready. The Golden Hour is a standard that all hospital trauma centers follow when it comes to shooting and trauma. If you can stabilize the patient and get them into surgery within an hour, the chance of recovery is extremely high. I had no problem taking a life to protect my team. I had a combination of lifesaving medication and the most advanced weapons of the time. My weapon of choice to take into the hot zone was the Heckler & Koch MP5 submachine gun. With the thumb switch next to the trigger, I could click between single shot, 3-round burst, and fully automatic.

I had a drug box in the trunk of my vehicle and was on call 24/7. The guys on the SWAT team were fit, smart, and a definite cut above. Instead of standing still in front of a target, we would have to run full speed, stop, jump over a barrel, and then shoot straight with a heart rate of 160 bpm. In my mind, I said, *Hell, yes! This is training for reality!* This was much needed—and appreciated—by my brain, which craved dopamine.

Working as a SWAT medic full time did not interest me in the least, but my interest in physical performance kept me fascinated. I still had a passion to learn more about the interconnected systems of metabolism, namely the behaviors and diets of my team members. How we dealt with family and friends while under stress was going to be an important topic in a few years. A new field of science called psychoneuroimmunology, which basically says, "Show me your friends and I'll show you your health," was on the horizon. People would come to realize its critical importance in the near future.

This was 1984, and I was also training for the St. Anthony's Triathlon in Tampa, Florida. Most of the SWAT team knew that I was a triathlete, as they would see me training in the city, so they were open to experimentation. We would do interval training on the track, running repeat loops of 400 meters as fast as we could with a heart rate of 180 bpm and then resting until our heart rates dropped to 100. The speed at which your heart rate dropped determined your fitness.

There were no physical fitness requirements while I attended the police academy, which needs to change (along with adding psychological profiling). The obesity rate in police officers is double that of the general public. Being hyperalert 24/7, 365 days a year blocks the arteries faster than a three-pack-a-day smoking habit. When you add in the low testosterone and growth hormone from elevated cortisol, this cuts life expectancy in half.

The reality no one talks about was that if you chase a bad guy for three minutes, flat-out, with a heart rate of 180 bpm, and then draw your weapon and fire, you will most likely miss the bad guys and hit a citizen. As we moved from the Smith & Wesson six shooters to the Sigs, it took months of training at the range before the gun became an extension of my arm again. Whether it's a hockey stick, baseball bat, golf club, or automatic weapon, you have to stay on it every day to be the best.

At that time, I was in contact with Brian Maxwell, who developed the PowerBar with his wife in his home kitchen. He was looking for something to eat before he went running that would not upset his stomach, and *voila*, the PowerBar was born. He later sold it to Kraft for a cool $144 million. Brian sent me a few boxes of PowerBars for the SWAT team. Not understanding metabolic pathways as I do now, I gave the guys the PowerBars on a stakeout to maintain their energy. Big mistake, as half the team almost fell asleep due to the sugar crash. Most of the SWAT team, and triathletes like myself, were addicted to carbohydrates. Many of us had to eat every three to four hours, which was killing us softly.

This is where I started to notice how caffeine and nicotine enhanced my brain chemistry. I would always eat a PowerBar before going to the range, which spiked my insulin and blood glucose levels. I would crash an hour into training and get the shakes, as well as brain fog. PowerBars were designed to be eaten while in motion, while riding a bike, for example. I then tweaked my diet and began going to the range on an empty stomach. I would have two cups of black coffee with a cigarette to shut off my hunger. This protocol allowed me to focus; my reaction time went way down and my shooting improved almost immediately. I also felt good because of the dopamine burst. Nootropics (i.e., brain enhancement) was still twenty years away, but I was hacking my brain in 1984. I advanced this research when I became the Director of Research and Development at Signature Pharmacy—the Disney World of performance enhancement—but more on that later.

Between the emergency responder's lifestyle, the "collateral damage" of divorce, depression, and addictions, and the use of carbohydrates, alcohol, and drugs to deal with the dead air, it was only a matter of time before the body would start to shut down. Because of all the physical, mental, and emotional stress we all were under, we became extremely nutrient deficient.

When responding to emergencies, a little piece of you dies with each patient. These calls were starting to really bother me, but I kept my head down and kept moving forward. I knew I'd be out of there soon.

Chapter Five

FROM HERO TO ZERO

My mind was racing. I had just received notice from the Civil Service Board. After a lengthy legal battle for my job, I was terminated. Yep, that's right, fired! I was the first Lieutenant Paramedic in Winter Park to graduate from the police academy and be placed on the SWAT team. That might sound impressive, but in reality, my innovative ideas were constantly shot down, and I was viewed as a troublemaker. So much for going the extra mile! Sitting alone in my living room I kept thinking, *Wow, what the hell am I going to do now? This job is all I know; I will never make it as a civilian.*

Cognitive dissonance is the psychological stress of simultaneously holding conflicting beliefs in your head. I loved the job and the constant challenge of responding to emergency calls. No two were alike. None of that mattered, unfortunately, to those in power at the time. The political process is a nasty business, and I got caught in the crossfire during a very intense mayoral race.

I was pushing hard for change in the department, doing what was right to protect myself and my crew. I really didn't care who I pissed off. The fire chief, police chief, and city managers who ruled by fear and intimidation never got my respect. These obese, hormone-deficient, antidepressant-popping assholes needed to find another career.

It was clear the fire administration had built a paper trail on me with false allegations, and intimidation tactics were being used to get firemen to testify against me. We had hired four different fire chiefs over ten years, obviously an extremely volatile position. The whole thing was so disturbing for me that I couldn't sleep; I kept running scenarios in my head. I was worried about making money. I've always been somewhat entrepreneurial in my thinking, but that paycheck every two weeks was a sure thing. I was grinding my teeth so hard that I actually broke two molars and spit them into my hand one morning before my insubordination hearing. Be it the loss of a job or a family member, the metabolism from your brain to your gut is working overtime and you're on that damn hamster wheel—and good luck trying to get off.

As I look back, this was the best thing that could have happened to me. People dying, the lights, sirens, being hyperalert 24/7... I was done. My body and mind were breaking down, and I would swing between rage and elation. I even stood on the steps of city hall and defiantly yelled at the city manager, "You fucked with the wrong person! It ain't over, motherfucker!"

That was a rage day. If you would have told me that in just a few years I would be interviewed by Mike Fish of ESPN and David Epstein from *Sports Illustrated* as a performance enhancement expert who was working with professional athletes and celebrities, I would have said, "No way in hell."

It took my pension of $40k to hire an attorney. I testified against the police chief in a sexual harassment investigation. I also testified against the city manager and fire chief. Less than twelve months after my termination, all involved were let go or fired. Mission accomplished. I really didn't care about the people who tried to ruin my life. I was told my case cost the city two million dollars.

I was devastated by the termination; my life was all about rescuing people and using my unique skill set. I didn't care about the money; it was how I felt when I restarted someone's heart. It was a rush and a feeling that carried me for days. I was one of the best, thanks to Dr. Corvelli and Dr. Wurtzel, my mentors at Winter Park Hospital; I would see signs and symptoms before anyone else. Other paramedics would say, "Teach me," but I never knew how.

It was just very clear to me when I'd sit next to a patient and get their medical history. This all had to take place in minutes. With each emergency call, each patient, my ability was amplified. Responding to ten emergency calls a day, I got my 10,000 hours in a few years on the job. Losing all that was overwhelming, and because I was a lieutenant, a go-to guy, I had no one to talk to on the job. This is where my father's voice resonated in my head. When I was a kid, he would drip science and psychology on me with stories. Somehow, he knew I would remember the stories during the times life kicked my ass. He would say, "Russ, remember, when it comes to people, if you're swimming they'll swim with ya; if you drown, you drown alone."

They say American Indian warriors never suffered from PTSD after years of battle because they went back to hunting and caring for the community. This gave them a sense of purpose. I lived with triathletes; we were all together most of the time. The stress of my legal battle with the city was offset by my tribe of warriors, or at least that's how I wrapped my brain around it. I was so proud to be able to watch and train with these people; they all were truly gifted. I was super curious and excited to race. I was training full time. I also enrolled at Rollins College to pursue my bachelor's and master's degrees.

My new community kept me healthy, focused, and jacked into a sport many people didn't even know existed. Again, I was with a group that was one of the first to explore this swim, bike, and run competition, imagining someday to be competing in the Hawaiian Ironman. This much-vaunted death march consists of a 2.4-mile ocean swim, a 112-mile bike race, and a 26.2-mile marathon, a race only a rare few could ever even think about completing. I wondered, what was the metabolism doing at five hours into a race with an average finishing time of 15 hours? I was entering a new world of research, and using my understanding of physiological pathways to study and enhance performance was another golden opportunity.

This allowed me to exhale from all the mental trauma. Responding to emergency calls is like playing contact sports—your time in the game is limited. From the first emergency call you respond to, an internal fuse is lit and it's just a matter of time before you blow up. We all medicated our brain chemistry with simple carbohydrates and alcohol on our days off. There was no testing for brain chemistry in the early days, but I knew from my own research that elevated cortisol damages a part of the brain called the hippocampus, which processes short-term memory. I was beginning to have trouble with short-term memory and kept blowing it off.

As I increased my triathlon training, being outside in the sun for hours had a healing effect, elevating my serotonin levels. We fell into a routine where we would all go to bed around 9:00 pm, get up at 5:00 am, and hit the pool for a 3,000-yard workout. We would go to breakfast as a group. I missed my community of firemen, cops, and paramedics, but the transition to a new community of people was seamless. As a community of athletes, when we were injured— mentally or physically—we supported each other. I thought about military basic training. From the start, men and women are within five feet of each other when they eat, sleep, train, and go to battle. But military vets are sent home alone. They lose their community. And we wonder why there are so many suicides and addictions among our vets.

I ended up diving into performance enhancement around this time as well. Endurance athletes were in a constant state of muscle wasting, or sarcopenia. The proper ratios of fats, carbohydrates, and proteins were on our minds unceasingly. The book *The Zone* by Barry Sears was on the best-seller list and all the triathletes were reading it. What were the best supplements for recovery? Hundreds of hours were spent on how vitamins, minerals, and amino acids affected metabolism. Sarcopenia also happens to AIDS and cancer patients. I studied their diets, drilling down on how physicians at the time were helping them maintain muscle mass. Testosterone and growth hormone were extremely important; both these hormones are suppressed with elevated cortisol.

The idea of training and testing endurance athletes was highly appealing to me. This distracted my attention from the devastating loss of a job I truly loved. It kept my intensity levels elevated without the lights and sirens. I had to stay in motion. As long as I was moving, my mood was fine. It's the dead air, the downtime when you're alone where you can get into trouble. I had my friends who still loved me. Now I had a new quest, another mountain to climb. Maybe through helping athletes I could find the same gratification I got from saving lives.

I was also in grad school meeting people and professors who became my mentors. I knew I wanted to continue to help people, but was not sure where I should apply this skill set. I was not going back to emergency work; it was time to just train and study. The research on the endurance athletes and bodybuilders provided me with an intense understanding of human metabolism on a cellular level. Meeting and talking with these people allowed me to witness their culture.

While in grad school, I wrote a paper on the aging work force. Standard operating procedures change as technology and testing allows people to work until their 70s, 80s, and 90s. Everyone thinks retirement is a party; it's actually a trauma for many people who lose their community and their self-worth. I thought I could focus on this area; maybe this could make a difference versus working on 300-pound cardiac arrest victims. If I could catch these folks early with nutritional and hormonal support, I could improve their quality of life. Since I was a kid, I had always wondered why some people in their 60s looked and acted so young. If I could break that down, I could be on to something—and be the first out of the blocks with it. The idea intrigued me, and I've always loved a challenge.

Chapter Six

DRIPPING THE SCIENCE

I've learned that every culture has its artifacts and heroes, and there is no swaying its thinking. It's a religion. The skill is to listen and slowly drip science that will assist in changing the current belief system.

As a result of my passion for saving lives and my background in biochemistry and physiology, I started testing athletes. As a paramedic, I'd responded to heart patients and corrected deadly arrhythmias. I would see these same arrhythmias even in super-fit individuals. This was the ideal foundation for me to make a real difference in cardiovascular treatment in the years to come. Anytime you bridge the gap between two cultures that don't communicate—like emergency service professionals and endurance athletes—you see things before everyone else. Years later, I would be training cardiologists and making discoveries that no one could believe, but at that time, I just wanted to stop drinking and hang out with a different group of people.

I got to travel to Metametrix, a lab that provided testing to identify nutritional imbalances and toxicities, in 1995 and met the owner, Alexander Bradley, as well as nutritionist Terry Pollock. My goal was to test endurance athletes in order to track nutritional and hormonal deficiencies and then correct these deficiencies to increase performance and speed recovery.

Alec Rukosuev was the first pro triathlete I tested. Alec was from Russia, barely spoke English, and was so fast that I knew he could win the Ironman one day. I tested Alec on a cellular level with advanced nutritional and hormonal labs. It showed elevated cortisol levels and a deficiency in gamma-linolenic acid (GLA), which is an omega-6 fatty acid. I thought instead of giving athletes liver-damaging anti-inflammatory drugs, we could use a balance of safe essential fatty acids that could protect the adrenal glands and speed recovery in these athletes. This was fascinating because there was no research in this area of metabolic imbalances. For me, this was like saving lives as a paramedic; with this testing, I could lead the way in performance and recovery.

In 1998, I visited a research lab called Atherotech. There I met with Kenneth French, PhD, the Chief Lipid Science Officer. This was the first company to develop the VAP test, the Vertical Auto Profile. They understood in the early 1990s that cholesterol was not the only cause of heart disease. More specifically, their testing looked at lipid subfractions. Think about cholesterol as a big beach ball floating around in our blood. There is a cholesterol subfraction that is much smaller than a beach ball, more like the size of a marble. Atherotech and the research done by Dr. French shows that this "marble" is a repair protein, a smaller form of cholesterol that could pass into the lining of the arteries and start blockages. The mistake being made by conventional cardiologists was pinning heart disease solely on cholesterol. Heart disease is a multifactorial disease process. The other mistake was looking at total cholesterol when only the damaging subfractions needed to be considered.

I spoke to Dr. French for hours and met the staff. Finally, I was getting justification for my beliefs. Thankfully, these people I met along my journey to becoming a high-level interventionist kept me focused and never allowed the thought of quitting to enter my mind. I was over the hyperalert brain-draining culture of emergency services and, like any explorer of the past, I needed to set my ship on another course. I knew that I would enjoy this new adventure too, since I was approaching it with the same fascination with the human metabolism that I'd always had as a kid.

I was on the fast track, a man on a mission. When you feel it in your gut, it becomes an obsession, which can be a good thing if it keeps you focused on your goals. I traveled to the best research labs in the country and met leaders in the field of advanced metabolic testing, absorbing information like Luke Skywalker from Yoda.

Following my instincts and the facts, I became more convinced than ever that the current treatment for heart disease, diabetes, and obesity was all wrong, but who was I? And who would actually listen? There is a Far Side comic that fittingly illustrates my life. There's a guy with a camera and standing right in front of him is Bigfoot, the Loch Ness monster, and a UFO—and then his camera jams!

Throughout the history of medicine, anyone who has made amazing discoveries was shot down by their peers, most of whom were too lazy or inept to break any new ground themselves. I understood this, but still moved forward, knowing in my heart and mind that the current heart disease treatment was wrong. Thousands of cardiologists across the world were telling people that fat caused heart attacks, but they were wrong. Emergency service personnel, cops, firemen, and paramedics have the highest heart attack rate of almost any line of work, even though their diet isn't significantly worse than the rest of the population. What was the explanation for that?

It was clear to me that heart disease, the actual blocking of the coronary arteries, had to come from multiple areas. The advanced testing I was putting together carefully studied these areas for the first time with endurance athletes having these same coronary artery blockages. I had to peel the layers off the onion and find the sweeping generalization that tied emergency personnel with endurance athletes. What did they have in common? I already had the research that very effectively demonstrated how physical, mental, and emotional stress causes elevated cortisol and low testosterone. Forget about muscles and libido for a second; from a heart disease perspective, testosterone protects the arteries by helping release a gas called NO (nitric oxide) from the endothelial lining of the walls of the arteries. This process dilates the coronary arteries that surround the heart, allowing lifesaving oxygen and nutrients to feed the myocardium, i.e., the heart muscle.

When emergency workers or endurance athletes come under stress, which results in elevated cortisol levels, the exact opposite happens; the arteries constrict because the body is in fight-or-flight mode. Both low testosterone and high cortisol lead to restricted arteries, a one-two punch. This chronic stress and its physiological effects on the body, over time, is what causes heart attacks, **not just cholesterol.** In fact, every human needs cholesterol to make every hormone in the body, including testosterone. It is sad that we have made people afraid of cholesterol, a vital substance.

Stress isn't the only thing that contributes to heart disease. While responding to heart attack, stroke, and diabetic emergencies, I noticed most of the patients were obese. Diet elevates blood glucose and insulin, the fat-storing hormone, which obviously played a major role in all these conditions. Why then, with 4,000 hours of training to become a physician, are *zero* hours spent on diet and nutritional support?

That is an outrageous state of affairs. I would get awards for saving lives, but in reality, these people would go back to eating the standard American diet, which is far too high in carbohydrates. Consider this: you have about 1,000 teaspoons of blood circulating in your body… and 1 teaspoon of sugar. The American diet is way too high in sugar. This seemingly innocuous white powder is a main contributor to heart disease, not fat, as everyone has thought for decades. The endurance athletes may have been lean and fit, but they were doing the same damage to their bodies by loading up on carbohydrates for training and racing. All of us drank the Kool-Aid, but there was no other way to say it: the current treatment protocols for heart patients were wrong. How did we as a country get this so wrong? Why did we blame cholesterol and fat for heart attacks when the research shows that carbohydrates and high insulin can begin blocking the arteries when we are children? Fat was not the cause of heart attacks; it was the carbohydrates.

It sounds like a conspiracy, but it started in the 1950s with a guy named Ancel Keys, who said that his research showed that heart attacks were caused by high-fat diets. This misinformation went viral and we are still paying for it to this day. Billions were made on cholesterol-lowering drugs with slick marketing for physicians and the public. We were convinced that cholesterol was bad and focused on our good and bad cholesterol. In reality, this was all based on misinformation… but try explaining that to a cardiologist. Cardiologists will call you crazy. I realized, of course, that it would take years for this new thinking to go mainstream.

There was a double-blind clinical trial on a cholesterol-lowering statin drug that the FDA deemed safe, which meant nothing to me. The list of folks I responded to who had severe reactions from just taking normal doses of the medicine was long and distinguished.

The athletes I knew who were taking statins would get pain in their legs and have to back off their weekly training mileage. Other people would get brain fog, and because I lived and trained for hundreds of hours with these people, I would often listen to their complaints. The heart is a muscle, and that muscle needs energy, nutrients, and oxygen. Statins damage that process on a cellular level. The PhDs at the research lab told me in the 1990s that statins block CoQ10 inside the mitochondria. With CoQ10 blocked, the cells are not able to create energy. When this research was shared with me, I couldn't believe it. On top of that, cholesterol is needed to make every hormone in the metabolism. The trillions of cells in the body are surrounded by a lipid bilayer that is made from cholesterol. How could there be such a thing as bad cholesterol?

Restarting someone's heart and bringing them back to life is an extreme rush, particularly knowing that it was your hands and your quick thinking that made it happen. Only those who have experienced this will know the feeling. However, in the back of my mind, I knew that these people I saved would revert to eating bad, smoking, and drinking. Did I really save a life or merely prolong a shitty existence? How could I save lives the way I wanted to? I came to realize that I would have to start working on prevention programs, because if I truly wanted to save people, it had to start much earlier.

Testing blood levels on athletes revealed that the combination of training and elevated cortisol lowers all the hormones: testosterone, thyroid, and growth hormone. I found that the large amount of carbohydrates consumed by endurance athletes was causing cellular damage, as well as yeast overgrowth in the gut. Having the correct balance of intestinal flora is essential to performance and recovery. Plus, mitochondria burn fats more efficiently than carbohydrates with less "smoke" or free radical damage. By eating a high-carb diet and training and racing these distances, endurance athletes were accelerating their aging process through something called oxidative stress.

To see this in action, cut an apple in half and spray one side of the apple with lemon juice. You will see the other half of the apple getting brown. That's oxidation. The side of the apple sprayed with the lemon juice stays fresh; this is an example of the antioxidant protection from the vitamin C in lemon juice. When pounding the carbohydrates and high-sugar sports drinks, I was releasing bursts of free radicals, causing oxidative stress; this was browning my vital internal organs, like basting a turkey. The pain and inflammation were unbearable, but I pressed on, thinking that fast race times meant I was healthy. I was so wrong.

Once I started training over longer distances, I was curious about how far and how fast I could go. My education in biology and human metabolism gave me a unique skill set in terms of hacking performance. My ability to shut off the pain was both a gift and a curse. I kept a training diary to track food, sleep, race times, and recovery. After a long, fast bike ride of 75 to 100 miles, my legs would recover in about two to three days, but my heart would not, and I needed to take more time off.

Every time your heart beats, the force is equal to lifting 70 pounds one foot off the ground… how about that for a muscle? The ejection fraction is the percentage of blood pumped out of the left ventricle with each contraction. This measurement helps determine how well your heart is functioning. The hearts of some athletes have a very low ejection fraction, indicating their hearts never have a chance to recover. The heart is a muscle that no one thinks about after long training and racing seasons. Almost all athletes focused on how their legs felt after long training days. I knew this was not a good indicator of recovery.

Most physicians don't understand an athlete's metabolism, and they sure as hell don't understand the damage that training and racing can do. And it's not just the heart that gets damaged. For example, the position of a cyclist, bent over on the racing bike, combined with an extremely high heart rate, can cause poor circulation to the intestinal tract. Some cyclists have been forced to have part of their intestinal tract removed. This bent-over position can also cause small blood vessels to bleed, leading to a subclinical anemia not found in blood tests.

When a runner's foot strikes the ground repeatedly for 26.2 miles, the distance of a marathon, red blood cells start to break apart. This is called foot strike hemolysis. This slows recovery from training and racing, and is missed by most of the "Dalai Lama" exercise physiologists in the performance arena. The blood tests of athletes always confused physicians; their blood tests were normal, but they complained about depression, mood swings, and fatigue. They simply didn't look sick—indeed, they looked tan and fit and had a low resting heart rate; but they were very sick.

The testing we did looked at the athletes on a cellular level. I looked at how well the athletes were breaking down carbohydrates, fats, and protein to make ATP, the energy currency of life. We were also able to test for nutritional deficiencies inside the mitochondria, which was mind-blowing. The mitochondria are the little batteries in every cell of our body, and we have trillions of them. Mitochondrial dysfunction is the starting point for most diseases.

In the nineties, I did extensive research, met with athletes having bizarre symptoms, and then handed their physicians the data I'd collected in order to get the athletes help. The physicians totally disregarded the research. This was maddening to me, to say the least.

My payback came years later when my job consisted of training physicians in nutritional and hormonal health, but at that time, it was like chipping away at an iceberg with a toothpick. The arrogance of those physicians was annoying as hell and made no sense to me.

This dogma, combined with the automaton-like, conformist thinking of the American Medical Association, is literally killing people. That is one more reason why, from early on in my research, I have videotaped patients explaining their health in their own words, as I believe this is one of the best ways to educate the masses.

Racing, training, and living with endurance athletes and working with the SWAT team, all while traveling to the most advanced research laboratories in the country, helped me drill down on the metabolic puzzle pieces of performance enhancement. I had knowledge of hacking the heart and administering lifesaving drugs on emergency scenes. However, I had to combine this knowledge with my recent discoveries in the area of nutritional biochemistry. The big difference between vitamins and food is that synthetic vitamins don't have cofactors (enzymes and other substances that haven't been discovered yet) that allow your body to absorb nutrients in food. Knowing this helped me avoid buying into the slick marketing of the billion-dollar vitamin industry. Think about it. You are not what you eat, but rather, what you absorb.

In the 1990s, we learned how to maintain muscle mass by following the bodybuilder community. But the bodybuilder community didn't understand that, as they were building extra muscle, they were ignoring (and damaging) the heart. As an endurance athlete, it was about being strong and lean, with a focus on the heart and a healthy circulatory system. Adults have almost 100,000 miles of veins, arteries, and capillaries that bring nutrients and oxygen to the muscles. That is tough to wrap your head around, the concept that any extra muscle was basically not needed if the circulatory system was healthy. Climbing a mountain in the Tour de France, you have to be as light and strong as possible, and you must have the right level of hemoglobin and hematocrit. These blood markers determine the amount of oxygen-carrying red blood cells. The more red blood cells, the less lactic acid in the muscle, and the better performance and recovery. The reason cyclists take erythropoietin (EPO) is to increase red blood cells and the nutrients and oxygen they provide to the cells. This is the same reason they use their own blood in transfusions, to increase the oxygen-carrying capacity of the blood cells; cheating will continue as long as sport exists.

I realized that the lab tests we collected on athletes would help heart attack victims recover. Keep in mind that no cardiologists at that time ever considered nutritional and hormonal replacement for recovery. I knew I could change the paradigm. This is why I started the Institute of Nutritional Medicine & Cardiovascular Research. I knew we had to open source this research for the public. Soon, every heart patient will be on a high-fat diet combined with micro-doses of testosterone. I have trained hundreds of physicians on the lifesaving effect of testosterone. Forget libido and muscle and think about neuroplasticity, synaptogenesis, and neurotransmitter levels, as well as heart function. Testosterone allows the arteries around the heart to stay wide open, including the left anterior descending artery, which when clogged, causes the highly fatal widow-maker heart attack.

One of the programs we eventually developed was an antidepressant withdrawal program. No one knew back then that antidepressants were addictive and could damage the mitochondria on the cellular level. Testosterone was part of the first-line treatment protocols because of its effect on the feel-good neurotransmitters. Again, doctors would enter my office with a swagger and leave humbled. I never wanted to make enemies; I saw every meeting with physicians as a time to educate and brainstorm ideas, with helping patients as the number-one goal. Many physicians would say, "Russ, I love your program, but I have to see 40 people a day. I just have no time."

The number of physicians that shut the door in my face is too many to count. The arguments and the name-calling were just uncalled for. All I was doing was trying to help people get answers—answers I'd already researched—and this frustration kept my fires burning. For any of you reading these lines, if you have a basic understanding of human metabolism, no physician will ever be able to lead you down the wrong road again.

The research on endurance athletes and bodybuilders pointed me in the right direction. I was helping people with specific diseases that cause muscle wasting: cancer, HIV, and sarcopenia (muscle wasting in the elderly).

When the metabolism becomes deficient, the body will mine nutrients from the bones and muscle tissue. In order to run the human machine, the average person needs daily 21 minerals, 13 vitamins, 8 amino acids from protein, 2 essential fats, and some sunlight to kick-start the whole process. If these nutrients are not absorbed from food, the metabolism will mine these nutrients from the body. When you hit level 4 REM sleep, growth hormone is released. Growth hormone is also called the repair hormone, and needs nutrients to rebuild the body. This is where food and hormonal replacement in the right combinations can save your life.

Performance enhancement has been around since the beginning of time and it's not going away. People are buying steroids online, not doing the correct blood work, getting into trouble, and throwing blood clots... brilliant. With just a little research, they can advance their health, maintain their heart and brain, and live to see 100... easily. This became so clear to me after taking people into nursing homes and watching them deteriorate. I then watched the exact opposite happen with people in their 70s at anti-aging centers by optimizing hormonal levels—they were still healthy and active.

My hard head and passion to keep asking questions kept us out front in the performance enhancement arena. Once people understand the basics of biological systems—which, when taught correctly is not hard to understand—they make informed decisions about supplements. Think about the guys with extreme muscle mass advertising whey protein on the cover of *Men's Muscle* magazine; that's fake, if you catch my drift. Is it any secret that these well-muscled men are on the juice? Muscle is very expensive to maintain, but I'm not judging. I have learned as much from bodybuilders about muscle development as I've learned from endurance athletes and cancer patients about muscle wasting. I can tell you that I've sat next to the best physicians in the country and showed them the research that we gathered from these outliers, and they are always amazed. Many have become my partners.

While athletes around the country were swallowing hundreds of dollars' worth of supplements they didn't need, I was testing for nutritional and hormonal deficiencies. These tests and treatments kept evolving every year. We started in 1984. Think about that for a second... we were the first group of athletes to use a high-fat diet in 1996. Then in 2016 the ketogenic diet for athletes became the hottest and most controversial topic on the planet; the grain industry stands to lose billions when people start eating more fat and fewer carbs.

The history of the high-fat diet goes back thousands of years. Indigenous tribes like the Maasai, Aborigines, and Inuit all had diets that were low in carbohydrates and high in fat. Evolutionary biologists tracked the diet and health of these people, comparing the benefits to the standard American diet and the obesity epidemic. There are people around the world who understand this research, and while they may not be well known or on the front of *TIME* magazine, trust me, they are flying under the radar. People are saving lives every day using high-fat and low-carbohydrate diets as the foundation of fighting disease. The worldwide implications are extraordinary.

Chapter Seven

SIGNATURE PHARMACY BUSTED

Signature Pharmacy will forever be known for its role in the biggest steroid bust in US history. This is the backstory.

I started the Institute of Nutritional Medicine & Cardiovascular Research, LLC, to pull together the research on why ultra-fit endurance athletes were having heart attacks and arrhythmias, with the ultimate goal of helping regular folks with heart disease. Scott Levitt, a good friend, was the first person for whom I created a treatment protocol. Scott's story is on the Russ Scala YouTube channel, and we still use Scott's program to educate cardiologists today.

I was at the foot of Scott's bed in CCU with the research in my hands for the cardiologist, right after Scott hit the ground with chest pain. All the physicians who were called were at a loss about what to do. Scott was ultra-fit, and I was training and racing with him. His resting heart rate was in the low 40 beats per minute. He had a head of steel during hill workouts and could always push through the pain. This is what separates athletes with equal skills; it's always who has the head, the focus and the ability to detach from the pain and keep moving forward.

The arrogance of cardiologists was just part of doing business. I understood the fact that these guys made hospitals billions in revenue with heart bypass surgeries. At $80k a pop, everyone kissed their ring and ass at the same time, including hospital administration. In a short time, every cardiologist on the planet will come to realize all the harm that they did recommending low-fat living. As I've stated, research has shown that cholesterol is one of the most important nutrients in the metabolism, and that there is no such thing as bad cholesterol. Billions—with a B—were made on cholesterol-lowering drugs, which will be one of the biggest lies ever perpetrated by the medical field on the American people.

I established a partnership with a molecular research lab and got Scott set up on some advanced cellular testing. We looked at all his nutritional and hormonal deficiencies, as well as the high-fat, low-carbohydrate diet. Scott's symptoms were not from high cholesterol, but from multiple nutritional and hormonal deficiencies. The perfect storm that blocked his arteries was elevated cortisol and insulin, which suppressed his thyroid gland and reduced his testosterone levels. Testosterone in the right balance protects the lining of the arteries, called the endothelial lining. If an athlete keeps training with an elevated heart rate between 160 and 180, the endothelial lining becomes damaged and a repair protein is released. It's like covering a hole in a wall of your home with spackle; that spackle is what blocks the arteries. Scott had a stent surgically inserted into his blocked artery to keep it open, but this procedure alone can damage the artery and cause restenosis, the recurrence of abnormal narrowing of an artery or valve after corrective surgery. The insertion of a stent can save the life of a heart attack victim, but because the placement of the stents damages the endothelial lining, it can become reblocked.

What I developed for Scott was a program that slowed restenosis. Scott's cardiologists prescribed the same meds that a 70-year-old would need: statins and blood thinners, neither of which he needed. As I mentioned, statin drugs cause a deficiency in CoQ10, a nutrient crucial to heart function. It is important to note that the testing we developed for Scott was not offered at any cardiology center in the United States at the time. Scott's program, and the video about it, has saved hundreds of lives for those who believe the research.

The next day, I was on a 25-mile bike ride with the group, and riding next to me was Kirk Calvert. Kirk was a buddy who had just started working with a new pharmacy in Orlando. I was telling him about Scott's nutritional program. Kirk asked me if I would like to meet the owners of the pharmacy, Stan and Naomi Loomis. I said, "Set it up."

That meeting set the next ten years of my life on a trajectory I could never have imagined.

Signature Pharmacy was in the business of bioidentical hormone replacement therapy. It was doing $5 million a year in revenue out of a small house that had been converted to a compounding pharmacy. Within three years, I would help them skyrocket to over $30 million in revenue, which led to a new $15-million-dollar, 10,000-square-foot pharmacy with my company as the research center. Just like a rags-to-riches movie plot, it was an exciting ride. When any company makes that much money that fast, it changes people.

I met with Stan and Naomi in their home and brought my colorful metabolism charts that explained the customized nutritional program I called E Juven 8. The testing I developed looked at eight metabolic systems, using blood and urine tests. I had the trademark, and after my presentation, the administration team said it was exactly what they had been looking for. No more going to GNC to buy supplements; this testing showed your exact nutritional deficiencies. The research showed that every person is biochemically unique and has different nutritional deficiencies. This program would develop an additional revenue stream with their existing distribution channel of 5,000 patients. The nutritional program was a perfect fit for hormone replacement. Compounding pharmacies across the US were also in the bioidentical business, but we would be the first to offer customized nutritional support based on results from a molecular research lab. I was already testing endurance athletes, which gave me a head start with educating physicians about this new program.

About 4,000 hours of training are required to graduate medical school, but zero hours are spent on nutritional and hormonal deficiencies and how they affect a patient's metabolism as they age. This was particularly exciting, because like the paramedic program, I would again be one of the first to roll out a new program that could potentially save thousands of lives.

I became the Director of Research at Signature, educating physicians on how multiple metabolic systems are involved in rehabbing heart patients and athletes. My company developed the first treatment protocol of its kind for a heart transplant patient. We looked at the new heart on a cellular level and measured its mitochondrial function—how the heart creates energy. All I could think about was, *Wow, this guy has a new heart belonging to another person, and I get to develop a program to keep him healthy!* This was a mind-blowing experience and I loved every second of it. This transplant patient is still with us today.

I agreed to the compensation package, which included a salary, a 20% commission on the product that went out the door with my company logo, and a black Porsche. I also had office space for the Institute of Nutritional Medicine and Cardiovascular Research. My cards said: *Russ Scala, Director of Research and Development, Signature Pharmacy.* We would travel from Orlando to New York to Vegas with physicians who were sponsored by the pharmacy. Drs. Sangeeta Pati and Claire Godfrey held seminars on bioidentical hormone replacement for men and women, and I would meet hundreds of physicians attending these conferences in each city. Signature quickly became the number-one pharmacy in the US, and word of mouth traveled fast about all the new programs we offered. Suzanne Somers, who has written bestsellers on hormone replacement, was saving the lives of thousands of women every day. Suzanne was often at these conferences educating people, and Signature Pharmacy was getting lifesaving bioidentical hormones into people's hands all over the US. We were all flying high.

When physicians had particularly complex cases, such as patients who were not responding to hormonal therapy, I would get a call and we would brainstorm what to do next—either increase the dosing or order more advanced lab tests. The physicians at the time were treating hormones in isolation, but the biology showed that all systems are interconnected. If a male is not responding to testosterone or growth hormone, or a woman is not responding to estrogen and progesterone, there are other areas to test.

Growth hormones became our best sellers, and within a year, I was contacted by David Epstein, a writer for *Sports Illustrated*. He said that he'd called five people in their New York office and asked, "Who is the number-one person in performance enhancement?"

David said to me, "Russ, your name came up all five times, and

I'd like to build a relationship with you." David went on to write the bestselling book, *The Sports Gene*.

I was soon tasked with developing blood work so that we could test a long-acting growth hormone. At the time, I thought that might be difficult, because billion-dollar pharmaceutical companies like Genentech had tried the same thing and had been unsuccessful, but I gave it a shot. We were testing people in-house with a small sample group, and did a rollout of long-acting growth hormone. Growth hormones and anabolic steroids got a bad name thanks to professional sports. It was never about muscle; it was about recovery. Athletes take a beating. The human metabolism makes steroids every day and as people age, they become hormonally deficient; they need steroids to stay healthy. Steroids protect the brain and heart of both men and women, but all the media talks about is the dark side. Steroids are naturally-occurring hormones in the human metabolism, but they were vilified by the media.

This was my first venture with a compounding pharmacy; the fact that they made and tested each medication for each patient fell in line with my research that concluded we are all biochemically unique. Big Pharma just generalizes a single medication for one disease condition. Hormonal deficiencies affect the heart, brain, and mental health, meaning that the list of what we could apply this treatment to was endless. While everyone else focused on libido and muscle mass, I was researching how hormonal deficiencies affect the big four: heart disease, diabetes, cancer, and obesity. I was also researching how traumatic brain injuries caused multiple hormonal deficiencies. Steroids would be needed to rehab war vets and people with strokes, as well as people with traumatic brain injuries. I met Dr. Mark Gordon in Vegas in 2006, and we had dinner together to discuss brain injuries and hormonal deficiencies. Mark went on to focus his work in this area. I knew that we could help thousands of emergency service personnel, athletes, and even war vets with this new and powerful research. The question was… how fast would it go mainstream?

Growth hormone was approved by the FDA in 1996 for adults with growth hormone deficiencies. Signature made it affordable for people at $500 a month. Big Pharma was charging $30,000 a year.

I developed blood tests to check insulin-like growth factor 1 (IGF-1). When IGF-1 was rising, we knew the growth hormone was working. However, there is a big trade-off between performance and longevity. Around this time, a few bodybuilders ended up with cancer. I remember their IGF-1, insulin, and blood glucose levels were through the roof. I thought this combination had caused the cancer; it was an inkling that would keep me awake at night. I knew that cancer metastasized in a high-glucose metabolism and that growth hormone raised blood sugar in some people. It was those people who used high doses of testosterone and growth hormones who got into trouble, but with the right dosage, growth hormone could save lives.

I was able to do research at Signature and develop new products that actually made a difference. Think about the weight-loss market for a second: calories and exercise never mattered. Allow me to explain… there are two enzymes that act like doors on the fat cell. Lipoprotein lipase is the door that allows fat into the cell to be stored, while hormone-sensitive lipase allows fat out of the cell to be burned as fuel. These doors are controlled by insulin, so if insulin goes up as a result of a high-carbohydrate diet, body fat increases. If a person keeps insulin down by cutting out the carbohydrates and increasing dietary fat, the person will stay lean. However, the billion-dollar weight-loss industry is not aware of this. Growth hormone elevates hormone-sensitive lipase, allowing people to burn fat very fast.

Weight loss is not about exercise. I have been testing endurance athletes for years who crossed the finish line after 26.2 miles and were still obese. It is not about calories, either. In fact, in some people, a half a slice of white bread will shut off fat burning for hours. Everyone metabolizes food in a different manner, depending on their hormone levels and intestinal flora. Fat distribution is under hormonal control; look at transgender folks, male to female or female to male. The muscle and fat distribution behaves in accordance with the exogenous hormone replacement that they are prescribed by their physicians. Estrogen distributes fat to a woman's breasts and buttocks, and testosterone alters the muscle-to-fat ratio with more lean body mass. Insulin and cortisol play a big metabolic role as well. The main takeaway is to correct hormonal and nutritional deficiencies and keep insulin levels low; that way, you will burn fat and keep muscle. This is where the ketogenic diet fits perfectly. I had the research and was ready to pull the trigger if I had access to the right facilities. This program would change weight loss for everyone.

I was light years away from responding to emergency calls, but in reality, I was doing much more; I was saving people *before* they got sick. With Signature marketing our program, we were going viral, which showed me how badly professional athletes and celebrities wanted my research on growth hormone.

My buddy Jason Bruce called from Infinite Vitality in Tampa, a hormone replacement center, and said that Jason Giambi, a superstar for the New York Yankees, was at their facility with some symptoms that were baffling the on-site physicians. Bruce asked me to design a customized performance testing and blood work program, and then send it to Infinite Vitality so they could test Giambi. When I received Giambi's test results, I explained why he was retaining fluid: his dosing of testosterone was way too high and he had elevated estrogen, as well as some nutritional deficiencies on the cellular level. Giambi needed to drop some body fat fast, so I tweaked the protocol, and Giambi responded well. While working with these clients, word of mouth traveled fast, like a brush fire. I was earning the title of performance enhancement expert; it's not what I considered myself, but I had to roll with it.

It wasn't long before physicians and athletes were contacting me from around the US, and shortly after designing Jason Giambi's protocol, I was in Vegas to meet Brad Friedmutter, the award-winning architect who built The Cosmopolitan of Las Vegas, the fifth-most expensive building in the world. Brad had offices in Las Vegas, Newport, Macau, and China, and I met his bodyguard, Joe, who was an ex-police officer. We became instant friends and he escorted me into the meeting with Brad and his team. I got the backstory on Brad's symptoms before the meeting from Joe, who had flown nonstop around the world with Brad in his Lear Jet. My history with the SWAT team and endurance athletes gave me a roadmap for how to help Brad. I thought, *Damn, with his support, we can do something really big.*

Once I got Brad feeling better, we met to discuss developing physician-based centers for the sick and famous inside the casino resorts. His CEO could never get his head around the business model, however, so the idea was pushed aside.

The reputation of Signature Pharmacy was gaining traction, though, and I was contacted weekly by venture capital investors about new and innovative ideas to change medicine.

Then one day, it all came crashing down. I turned on the morning news and saw a picture of myself and Dr. Claire Godfrey on a magazine cover that had been taken a few months earlier. Agents had entered Signature Pharmacy, locked down the facility, and arrested Claire. I was watching in shock, anticipating the knock on my door any second. Kirk, Stan, Naomi, and Mike were all similarly arrested and paraded out in orange jumpsuits on the six o'clock news. After the segment, my phone blew up. It was real, and it was getting national exposure. Within hours of seeing my picture with Dr. Godfrey on CNN, all I could think about was how fucked my life had just become.

The *New York Times*' lead story said that after a two-year investigation, federal and state investigators arrested four people with ties to Signature Pharmacy in Orlando for the distribution of tens of millions of dollars of performance-enhancing drugs. Celebrities were involved as customers and the four people were charged with criminal diversion of prescription medications.

My father's words again resonated in my head: "When you swim, they will swim with ya, but when you drown, you drown alone."

Everyone basically ran for the hills. My attorney even called and said, "Russ, I can't represent you."

I said, "Shawn, I haven't even been charged with anything."

The only person who came to my door was Scott Levitt. He said, "Russ, you were beside my hospital bed when I had my heart attack, so I'm here for you."

I put on my running shoes and headed out the door for a six-mile run. I needed to think about my next move. When I run, it slows down my brain, allowing me to drop screens in my mind and develop a plan. I had to get out of Orlando, so I headed to the beach for a few days. *If this investigation had been going on for two years, they have all my info and my cell phone number, so why haven't I been arrested?* Reporters and others from the media wanted me to give statements, but I had no idea what to say or not say. I had to go dark and think. The media circus continued for a few weeks, which is when one of my close friends, an attorney, called and said, "Russ, your name never came up. You are going to be fine. There have been no arrest warrants for you at all."

I started thinking… *Are you kidding me? All the research I developed, the new supplements, and working in synergy with the ketogenic diet was all lost?* I had new performance protocols for the high-fat diet and research on how it could help heart and diabetic patients, along with low-dose growth hormone and testosterone. I wanted to back up the files, but the computers had all been seized during the arrest. It was still hard for me to believe that everyone in Signature Pharmacy's administration had been arrested except for me. This led many to believe that I was working undercover due to my police and SWAT background. I had to put out a lot of fires. In the coming weeks, I was covered in kryptonite, and it took six more years before a judge exonerated Signature Pharmacy and all those who were arrested that day. The Feds' real problem was with the physicians who were prescribing and purchasing growth hormone for celebrities and athletes who were not deficient, which is illegal. Remember, growth hormone was FDA approved for adults with deficiencies only.

I had to keep moving and rebuild my reputation and my business, so I put my head down and focused on another distribution channel for my research. I had been through worse, but what saddened me the most was that we were right on the one-yard line with Signature, and we could have changed medicine forever.

Chapter Eight

AFTER THE SIGNATURE ARRESTS

I had to make some moves and make them fast. I was all over the national news for two weeks. My attorney advised me that I was in the clear, but I was still paranoid about people being wired and recording my conversations. With my SWAT background, I knew this was not paranoia, but a genuine concern. Whenever I met people, I always had my guard up, because they could be confidential informants, setting me up for prosecution. I trusted no one, and my girlfriend living with me at the time split right after the arrests; true love, right? This was not a good way for me to live. I needed office space, a physician, and a new pharmacy ASAP.

It didn't help the public's perception of me that I had transformed from a sick, 150-pound triathlete to 170 pounds of functional muscle running down Park Avenue for my daily workout. This metamorphosis led to whispers after the arrests. At 50 years of age, I had the body of a 30-year-old. Most 50-year-olds did not look like me; the testosterone, thyroid hormone, and growth hormone cut my body fat, which made my muscles really stand out. I would look in the mirror and not believe what I was seeing once I stopped the high-mileage training, decreased my cortisol levels, and let my muscles come screaming back. People who watched me run around the city for years with the Winter Park Dawgs—a running group I started in 1996—looked at me and said, "Dude, what the hell are you doing?" This was not my goal, by any means, but I certainly wasn't disappointed. I had never felt that good in my life. What people don't realize is that it took three physicians and four years to rehab my metabolism. I was correcting nutritional and hormonal deficiencies that I'd had for years.

When I started growth hormone, I was scared. Before the injection, I stared at my lab tests that said I was growth hormone deficient. I knew that I needed this lifesaving medication, and I knew more about the research than anyone on the planet, but it was still hard to stick the needle under my skin. The way we tested if growth hormone was working back then was to check the IGF-1 blood marker. The range on the lab results goes from 100 to 300, and my labs showed my IGF-1 at 96. I was growth hormone deficient. The FDA had approved growth hormone for adults with this condition, and my goal was to get in the high two-hundreds. It took 90 days of injecting 1 IU of growth hormone every night, and as my levels increased, my sense of well-being improved 90%. Growth hormone and testosterone affect the feel-good neurotransmitters in the brain called dopamine. I had to get my lab tests every 90 days to stay on the program, and it was truly amazing. With all the stress in my life, I was in a good place and able to focus if I didn't exercise too much, because the elevated cortisol from exercise would simply stop all the benefits of the hormone replacement. I had to stay healthy because the only person taking care of me was me.

Wendy Chioji was a good friend and training partner. She was also the news anchor for WESH news, Channel 2 in Orlando. She was very public about her battle with cancer. I tested Wendy after she went into remission from cancer, and I developed a program for her before she did the Lance Armstrong ride for cancer in Texas. I found an elevated marker for cancer called 8 Hydroxy 2 Deoxyguanosine in her test results. This marker shows just how far ahead of traditional testing we were. This DNA marker, combined with elevated blood glucose and insulin from a high-carbohydrate diet, was the perfect storm for accelerating cancer growth and cellular mutations. I remember specifically telling her that she needed to change her diet and back off the training to lower systemic inflammation or the cancer would come back. Years later, it did.

Now Wendy is in a clinical trial trying to save her life. This has happened so many times with people who don't believe me. People do not understand that their physicians, despite their good intentions, are actually taking them down the wrong road. It is both frustrating and sad. What people do not realize is that cancer metastasizes in a high-glucose metabolism, so the ketogenic diet can be lifesaving, but getting people to believe that a high-fat, low-carb diet is safe is another story. We have all been conditioned for years to believe that fat is bad and causes heart attacks. This was dogma, but it was completely wrong. All Wendy had to do was change her diet and stop training at such a high level, but in her mind, how could exercise be bad?

I thought Wendy would put a positive spin on the Signature story, and she did reach out to me at the time of the arrest. However, I didn't know what I could say to the media, so I never called her back. She never did get the story, but I hoped people would forget in a few days and be on to the next media event. The public's short attention span was a good thing, in my case.

The hot topic, of course, was the celebrities and professional athletes. That is the kind of gossip that people like to talk about at the water cooler, and no one gives a shit about how true it is. The truth is boring, but performance enhancement in professional sports sells radio and TV time. People tuned in like it was a NASA shuttle launch.

I was quickly labeled as being part of the largest steroid bust in history, and no one was interested in the cutting-edge research I had done on heart disease, diabetes, or muscle wasting. They wanted to know about all the celebrities that were clients of Signature, so I had to find a new location for my company. I turned in the black Porsche for a Prius—*Ouch*—and I made a list of contacts I would reach out to. Looking over my shoulder and waiting for a knock on my door from the police kept me awake almost every night. The lack of sleep breaks your metabolism down fast, which I knew because of all my research. I had to adjust my own rehab program. When I am under stress, I start eating simple carbohydrates to get that bump of serotonin, which is a natural way to elevate my mood. I also incorporated brain nutrients, like 5HTP and GABA (gamma-aminobutyric acid); this combination with carbohydrates at night helped me get into REM sleep. The book *Potatoes not Prozac* speaks to this research. I had to dial back my training for triathlons; the mental stress of the arrests combined with the physical stress of training would simply be too much. Low-intensity training was the key that allowed me to still meet with my community of athletes. After any trauma, the people around you will determine how fast you heal. I stayed out of the bars and focused on getting a new location and pharmacy.

I had high-net-worth clients from around the US who needed my help and didn't care what the *New York Times* said, but I needed a location to meet them and a physician to write the prescriptions to rehab their metabolism.

I did lose some clients who bought into the media hype and, with them, it was a waste of time answering all the calls and putting out fires. People sometimes believed what they saw on the news. I could not control their thoughts.

I had the research on Alec Rukosuev, the professional triathlete, and was able to build a nutritional performance program that could help the intestinal tract absorb more nutrients from food. We were also using high-fat diet protocols and getting amazing results, but saying that we used a high-fat, low-carb approach made even the brightest PhDs in the country pass out. No one at that time was testing the gut. Remember, you are not what you eat, but what you absorb. I first focused on athletes as my new revenue stream. If you help the intestinal tract pull nutrients out of food more efficiently, their performance and recovery will be affected in a positive way. Here's the rub when it comes to the gut; it is critical to performance, rehab, and the prevention of disease.

As with all traumatic situations, there are people who pray for you, and people who just show up at your door. I had a few people I called friends, and the rest were just distractions I couldn't count on. I was used to a level of intensity with my work that was unimaginable to most people. When someone told me, "Russ, I got your back," in reality that meant these people were good for maybe one phone call. *How could you have my back when you have no idea what that means?* I wish I had a nickel for every time someone called me "intense." Whatever... I call it passionate. Kicking in doors and saving lives changes your view on life.

My family has 50 years of history in the City of Winter Park and the people who know me knew early on that I was not a criminal. Mike Fish of *ESPN The Magazine* flew in to meet me at Starbucks on

Park Avenue in Winter Park. I told Mike that every prescription that came to Signature came from a physician and that I didn't know what illegal activity had occurred. I trusted Mike as a top-notch investigative writer and believed that he would get the truth into people's hands. I explained to Mike that those same performance-enhancing drugs would soon be used to save lives and help our elderly population avoid heart disease, dementia, and cancer. We talked about the benefits of testosterone on a cellular level, and of growth hormone for congestive heart failure and dementia. I told him that the correct doses could improve injection fraction of the heart. The testosterone and growth hormone helped by making the myocardium stronger in people with congestive heart failure. I explained how I had worked on hundreds of patients with this condition as a paramedic, and I told Mike that if we got this into the hands of cardiologists, we could change the whole treatment approach for this terrible disease.

Mike asked about my research on growth hormone, and whether the long-acting growth hormone we developed at Signature was real and if it actually worked. I had to break down some biochemistry for Mike, helping him understand that physical, mental, and emotional stress activated the flight-or-fight response and elevated cortisol levels. When this happens, it shuts off growth hormone production like a light switch.

That said, each person is biochemically unique, so the dosing of growth hormone would be different in everyone. We could not simply make one dose for everyone. I also had to explain that growth hormone is just one part of an interconnected web of metabolic reactions, all of which have to be considered when you want to enhance performance or improve health. Bodybuilders that make the mistake of using super-physiological dosing are a good example of how other systems can break down. Maintaining twenty to thirty pounds of muscle mass is not healthy. Slick marketing makes people think that bulging biceps and six-pack abs equate to health, but it's actually the exact opposite.

Mike wanted to know if I had directly worked with professional athletes, and I said I had not. My direct contact was with physicians who needed research on bioidentical hormones, nutritional deficiencies, and growth hormones. Mike and I talked at Starbucks for about 90 minutes before he flew back to New York to write the story. I have kept in contact with Mike and shared all the research I've done since our meeting on the benefits of hormonal and nutritional replacement therapy.

I needed to find a new location to kick-start a new venture and get back on my feet after the Signature debacle. Dr. Sergio Mendez was in my running group, and he agreed to do the physicals for my clients who flew into Winter Park. Sergio had converted a small one-story house into a medical practice across the street from a pristine medical center. He spent time with each patient and understood the critical importance of nutritional support on the cellular level.

Sergio also knew my skill set and that I needed office space. I drove over to an imaging center called Specialty Imaging Service with no appointment, just walked in the door, and as luck would have it, Pam Bowen, the owner, remembered me from the days when I worked at Winter Park Hospital. I told Pam that I was building my business and she agreed not to charge me rent until I hit 25 new clients. The building was designed like a duplex; my side had a conference room and two small offices. It was not "high end" by any means, but it was all I needed. Pam had an iDexa imaging machine, where I could scan a patient and get their exact muscle-to-fat ratio. It was an amazing tool to help people with fat loss. When people check their weight by standing on a scale, it does not tell them their true weight. The scale doesn't say how much fat versus muscle a person has. This ratio is critical not only for performance, but also for disease prevention. People on a weight-loss program can lose muscle mass, but with this iDexa machine, I could avoid that and track it. Pam charged 100 bucks for the scan, which was perfect. I could scan a person and then hand off the results to a trainer to help them build muscle in the area of the body that was out of balance. I had a conference room with eight chairs to show my PowerPoint presentations, since I had to educate new clients on what their physicians were not offering. I had to drip the science slowly, so clients could wrap their heads around basic metabolism information and the ketogenic diet strategy.

Once the client agreed, I would set up advanced nutritional testing, and when the results came back, the client and I would meet Sergio at his office and develop a treatment plan. Sometimes I would have to sit in the waiting room with my clients for two hours, which was tough. I would explain all the advanced research and testing we did, and boast about how far we were out on the tip of the spear, only to sit and wait. However, I was grateful that I had two locations to kick off my program and get back on my feet.

Next up was Sam Pratt of Pharmacy Specialists. Sam was a good old boy with a Southern drawl. He has been in the pharmacy business for 30 years, and he had hired a few of the Signature employees. I needed Sam to close the loop on this business model, so he called Dr. Juanita Brown on a conference call. Dr. Brown was treating a woman who was in a wheelchair with an illness that was damaging her diaphragm, and she only had a few months to live. This was one of my first eleventh-hour interventions that put me on the clock; this was a time-sensitive protocol. I got that same rush as I once had on the emergency scene. I had no idea where else to go, so I took the case with the promise that Sam would fill the prescriptions written by Sergio for my clients. We came to a mutual agreement and over the next few weeks, I had to explain the programs I developed at Signature in detail. *Fair enough.* I pulled the trigger and went to work on this X-File case, and suddenly, I was back in business!

I would coordinate all the moving parts while educating the clients and giving talks around Winter Park at various locations and inside people's homes. There was both excitement and anxiety about starting over. I had a good team—Trent Duncan and Michelle Conti stepped up even when I could barely pay them—but that all would soon change.

People continued to hurl questions at me about the Signature bust, as well as the celebrities and professional athletes I had worked with. These people didn't care about me. Their lives were so dead and so boring that they just wanted the gossip, so I would avoid those leeches and hang out at Cigarz on the Avenue. The owner, Don Patel, had a back room that was off limits and open only to a select few people, making it the perfect location for me to decompress and regulate my brain chemistry. I didn't drink alcohol, but the nicotine had a calming effect on my neurotransmitter levels. To me, it was a drug, a natural antidepressant. Nicotine is a nootropic, and it's very interesting to study because it's a relaxant and a stimulant at the same time. They're still trying to develop billion-dollar drugs that have this effect. I've used nicotine with many of my high-functioning clients battling addictions as part of a nootropic treatment protocol. I also used nicotine for high-level code writers and Special Forces to help them increase situational awareness. There is new research on the combination of nicotine and caffeine slowing the progression of Parkinson's disease. When people think about nicotine, they instantly make the association with cigarettes, but that's a narrow way of thinking about it.

One of my clients arrived in his Rolls Royce, and when he got out of the car, I met him with a handshake and he started walking over to the new medical center. I had to say, "Marty, we're going over here," and pointed to Sergio's one-story building.

My client said, "Russ, are you kidding me?"

I replied, "Looks are deceiving. Trust me… I will get you the best treatment in the country."

This makes me laugh now; it was almost like a scene in a movie. Marty was in the medical field and owned a multimillion-dollar company and we are still friends today. My skill set was in helping get people answers. Many times, I would find the most complex symptoms in people challenging, but I would drill down with the advanced testing not offered through conventional medicine, which gave me a roadmap of their unique physiology. It was like trying to find a serial killer; I had to put many different puzzle pieces together. Many of these folks had been to four or five physicians with no answers, so by the time they met me, they were already mad and frustrated. I had to get them feeling better fast, so they would believe in the intervention.

Chapter Nine

THE IMPORTANCE OF THE BACKSTORY

One of the skill sets I developed over thirty years of being face-to-face with patients is finding the patterns hidden in chaos (like the bullet wounds obscured by the obvious car accident injuries). The physical, mental, and emotional stress of a divorce, a death in the family, a sick child, the loss of a job, or even an upsetting phone call can change a person's physiology and affect her health. The backstory is important. When I meet a new client, the Q&A helps me take a deep dive into her metabolism, along with administering some of the most advanced lab tests on the planet. I also have an understanding of the external factors that affect our health. This field of research is called social neurobiology. Basically, show me your three best friends and I will show you a picture of your health. That quote is easy to remember, and people repeat it when they hear it. It makes people think about their current situation, who is in their life, and how those people affect them.

Trudie Reed, a college president, came to me with a host of unexplained symptoms. When her test results came back, we found that her DNA was damaged. There was also a long list of nutritional and hormonal deficiencies. I told Trudie that we needed to check inside the walls of her office, as sick-building syndrome might have been the cause of her symptoms. Florida's damp weather is notorious for causing black mold to grow. Within a week, the office was tested and black mold was found. The building was evacuated and Trudie began to feel better within a few months. This was a big win for us without spending a dime on advertisement. Word of mouth was all I had. We helped a college president get answers when everyone else had failed.

Louis Amabile was Billy Badass before his brain injury. A proud guy and successful in business, Louis was on our nutritional and hormonal replacement program prior to his brain injury, and all his blood levels were at their peak. This is why Louis healed so fast after his motorcycle accident.

I knew his wife, his kids, and his friends, but his physicians had no idea what he was going through. Here's a guy who was bulletproof his whole life, but now, trying to focus on basic human functions like making a phone call was overwhelming to him. I knew that I had to target his depression specifically. If Louis became depressed, it would slow the rehab process. I'm not saying he had to have a party every day, but he had to feel as though he was making progress. This is what made him successful in business; I knew that the same mindset would help him recover.

That's precisely what we did. We tested his thyroid T3 levels and found that if we could optimize Louis' thyroid, it could help with his mood, energy, and brain rehabilitation. I didn't want Louis to take antidepressants, since those drugs are addicting and could damage his delicate neuronal cells. Fortunately, Louis had the drive and determination of a marathon runner. Each day, he had to dig deep and find the endurance to get through the hours. He really focused and studied what I sent him like a student going back to school. Except this time, he was getting a PhD in his own physiological functions. He had to stay in touch with me to make sure the treatments were working so I could call his physicians to adjust lab tests and tweak his dosing, if necessary. Louis' case was much more complicated than Trudie's, but what we learned helped us develop programs for traumatic brain injuries. Louis' before and after on the Russ Scala YouTube channel blew the hair back on neurologists who saw the transformation. My goal was to help traumatic brain injuries in war vets with this protocol.

Alan Castro was due to arrive at my office in ten minutes. Alan was one of the best cyclists in Orlando and was in amazing shape. He had trained for twenty years and rode hundreds of miles each week. Now he has the heart of another person beating in his chest, and he wanted to start over with his training. This was my first heart transplant case. I knew what tests to order, but I wanted to avoid going to battle with Alan's cardiologists, who knew nothing about the testing and rehab process that we were starting. I also understood that Alan had lost his community of cyclists. That alone is traumatic. The fact that he was extremely fit and his heart had failed him was a psychological issue that also had to be considered. How do you go from being one of the top cyclists in Orlando, racing with a team of eight, to becoming a regular citizen who has undergone a heart transplant? These guys are warriors; the dead air and downtime can kill them. When your metabolism is hardwired to ride hundreds of miles and recover, it becomes your life. When athletes halt their usual metabolic habits, it can lead to addictions to alcohol, drugs, or even food. I've witnessed this many times over the years with coworkers and training partners. It was the elephant in the room that no one ever discussed.

Alan seemed in good spirits and was already riding 20 miles a week with his new heart, a far cry from riding 400 miles, but you could see in his eyes that he was on the comeback trail. The focus, passion, and dedication of athletes always helps with their recovery. He understood that this would take time, but the very fact that he was back on the bike was exciting. My goal with this advanced research and testing was to correct all his nutritional and hormonal deficiencies and focus on performance and recovery while strengthening the new heart on a cellular level.

Again, the backstory is what helps my team create a treatment regimen that works. The traditional medicine that Alan's physicians were treating him with was like a single spoke in the wheel. These physicians had to see thirty people a day to pay the bills, which is where my team stands apart. We spend time with the patients, we educate the patient on where we are going with the treatment, and we encourage them to be an active participant in their treatment. How many cardiologists really appreciate a high-level cyclist when they're locked in a room all day writing prescriptions for cholesterol-lowering drugs?

I remember when Trudie called me late one night. When my cell phone rang and I saw it was her, I immediately knew that something was wrong. She said her personal physician called her and said that our treatment protocol was going to kill her. That's right… Trudie's physician said *we were going to kill her*! I thought, *Perfect, this guy is killing me*. This is very common, especially when physicians take care of celebrities or high-net-worth folks. There are bragging rights and a sense of "ownership" involved. These physicians look at me and say, "Who the hell are you? You're no doctor, and this is MY patient!" They don't want me on their turf and I get it… changing this situation always starts with a battle.

Usually, after a short conversation with these physicians, they understand what I do and see what they missed. Now their worry turns to liability. I always tell them, "Doc, you did the best you could, but you're not trained in this advanced research and testing."

Some physicians get pissed, but if they truly care about their patients, they roll with it. You would think that we all would work together, but that's much too rational. You would think that they would be open to getting another set of eyes on the situation. Eventually, after all that back and forth, I get respect and we can move forward. Remember, no physician will ever have all the answers, but most don't like admitting it. They continue to compartmentalize illness and injuries to one treatment regimen, rather than looking at the interconnected metabolic functions. One patient may have four different physicians prescribing medication, but these four physicians *never* talk to each other.

Physicians don't think about how the external environment causes hormonal dysregulation. The xenoestrogens from pollution are elevating all our estrogen levels, which leads to cell proliferation and cancer. When Trudie's hair began to fall out, the fact that her secretary had the same symptom was an immediate red flag for me.

I remember one family I worked with had a child with symptoms that five physicians could not figure out. It was the insecticides that were being sprayed around the house every month; the child's outbreaks were on a cycle. This is why the **backstory is so important** for me and my team to get answers. Every chemical a person rubs on their body—skin cream, toothpaste, antibacterial soap, shampoo, etc.—all of these can elevate estrogen levels. Once these chemicals are removed, the immune system can do a better job of keeping the body healthy.

Our medical system is not set up to take care of endurance athletes or the over-60 marathoners. Their numbers grow every year, and before long, having a productive quality of life past the age of 100 will be commonplace. You will see extremely fit 70-year-olds who want to train to climb K2, ride their bikes across Europe, and take on even more new and exciting challenges. Age is just a number to these people and they want to keep moving at any cost. Sitting in a recliner watching *The Price is Right* is worse than death to these people. Of course, I can relate.

This is where we are headed and I love it. The fact that I used to take people from their homes to assisted living centers while in their late 70s, and now I see amazing people still running road races in their 80s is mind-blowing! In my running group, called the Winter Park Dawgs, we have many runners who are over 60. I run with them every week and their mood, energy, and outlook on life is exceptional. I remember what my mother said to me after we brought her to stay at a daycare for older adults. I picked her up and asked, "Mom, how'd it go?" She said, "I'm not going back there. Those people are all old and all they did was talk about how sick they were." My mom was always active, walked five miles every day, and she was always in a good mood. In her mind, she was still young, so she wanted to be around young people.

This is my focus. If I can get people feeling better with these protocols, where they still have that gleam in their eye, maybe I can get this into assisted living centers—which we almost did while I was at Signature. Be it brain injuries or heart transplants, the surgery and recovery can be just as traumatic as the injuries. The field of research called psychoneuroimmunology, headed by Stanford PhD Dr. Sapolsky, shows us how even negative thoughts can lower the immune system. Just thinking bad thoughts or feeling that there is no way out causes a metabolic shift in the immune surveillance. The backstory on what a patient was doing prior to the incident is critical to the rehabilitation process.

Physical, mental, and emotional stress can lower a person's feel-good neurotransmitters, serotonin and dopamine. The goal during the rehab process is to keep these neurotransmitters as high as possible, which helps the healing process on the cellular level. Virtual reality headsets and mirror neurons will become a new paradigm of treatment. Research into mirror neurons has revealed that watching somebody take an action lights up the same part of the brain as actually taking the action yourself. This stimulates the development of new brain tissue, reinforcing the body's ability to take the action on its own.

There is one thing that I see with all these patients—once their rehab is over, they are left alone to fend for themselves, when in reality, the rehab can take years. My feeling is that if I can educate these folks on the Russ Scala YouTube channel, they can continue their rehab process by having their current physician get up to speed on the newest treatments available. These treatments are usually beyond the standard of care, so I have to work to get this new research into the hands of the real decision makers.

The key to data mining the backstory is to understand that patients have been told one thing by their physicians, while I'm showing them new research that says something completely different and making statements they may have never heard before. These people are scared and just want their lives back. Dripping the science slowly, gathering new research, and putting this complex data into terms they can apply and understand can take months, but the end results are astonishing. I've spent hours with four different physicians creating treatment protocols for these folks. Many times, I had to sit and wait to see physicians just to place the research into their hands; no one would come to my office because they were "too busy."

People still ask me, "Russ, why do you do this? Why go up against the medical system? Just let it go. It isn't worth your time."

What I do has never been about the money. I would regularly meet venture capitalists who drive up to the meeting in a Ferrari, pay for lunch with their black card, and pat me on the back, calling me a visionary. I never trusted these guys; most were just full of shit looking for the next big deal. These guys were always obese and on multiple medications. They were not healthy, but they wanted to get into the health business. I would look at them, knowing they were going to die screaming if they didn't make serious changes in their lives. To put it plainly, I was never impressed. Many of these guys were legends in their own minds. Because they were successful in one area, they thought they could be successful in the health arena. It never panned out; these venture capital guys we met were low level. They had a few bucks in the bank, a big house, a big mortgage. They were too comfortable to take risks and they lacked passion for changing the world. There are near-death experiences weekly with any startup and these guys would never last; they never had the endurance or fortitude. They wanted to build a company fast and then flip it. These types of people wasted hours of my time.

I've stood in front of beachfront mansions up and down the coast of Florida. I was always amazed. These people were so rich and so sick. You know what impresses me? A single parent who raises good kids while working full time. Now that's an accomplishment.

People with their withering remarks fail to realize that this is my passion, just like any artist. I do get obsessed with each client, but it's not nearly as bad as responding to emergency calls for 72 hours straight. Compared to the knife and gun club on South Orange Blossom Trail, this was a breeze. I knew what these people needed physically, emotionally, and metabolically. This kept me going. I also knew that I was on the road to new discoveries, which is exactly where I wanted to be.

Chapter Ten

MY CLIENTS, MY FAMILY

During an argument with a girlfriend one time, I was told that I was going to die alone because I never invested enough time into our relationship. That made me think about all the people who had died in my arms while we were rushing them back to the hospital.

I was the last person they saw before they passed. That thought would always hit me hard. Depending on the extent of their trauma, I always knew who would live and who wouldn't. I would just hold their hand while intravenous meds dripped into their veins to elevate their blood pressure, giving them a few more minutes of life. It is the memory of those situations that make me grateful I'm still standing after all these years. Truly, tomorrow is never a given.

All of my clients have my cell phone number and can call me 24/7 if symptoms or situations arise. If I need more lab work or have to adjust medication dosing, I contact our physicians on call. This way, the clients get help in real time without making an appointment and sitting in a waiting room with sick people for hours. Establishing a deep understanding of my clients helps me distill interventions that can get them feeling better sooner. So many of them have been feeling bad for years. A few of these clients have practically become part of my family, but that list is short. I've spent my life working high-intensity emergency scenes, and I had to put my life in the hands of people I trusted. In other words, my standard for friendship is high. I look at friendship like a target with the bull's-eye in the center; the outer, expanding rings of the target mirror the levels of friendships and acquaintances that I've made along the way.

The heart of the bull's-eye is where true friends reside. The people who say they've "got your back" really have no idea what that means. I truly don't expect anything in return from anyone. They often say to me, "We are here for you" or "We will pray for you." I've come to realize that these words are not meant for me; they are empty words that make *them* feel as if they have offered me some solace during a traumatic time. Do me a favor. Don't pray for me... that phrase is a cop-out.

The day I found both my mother and father dead in their home, two of my clients responded to me without hesitation, Erick Pace and Ricky Zabala. Ricky had to wait until the Cigarz store closed, but Erick arrived on the scene before the rescue crew even arrived and stood strong by my side. My mind was racing, trying to rationalize this extremely traumatic situation. I had responded to visually horrendous emergency scenes, but this day was worse than anything I had ever imagined. As I write these lines, I can still picture the position of my parents. It's extremely tough to deal with this kind of tragedy.

Word traveled fast in Winter Park. People avoided me because they didn't really know what to say. To those who said, "Russ, we're here for you, let us know if you need anything," my response was, "The funerals will cost about thirty-seven thousand dollars. Can you send money?"

That was followed by silence. My point is that 99.9% of people are full of shit, even those with millions in the bank.

Both Erick and Ricky started out as clients and evolved over the years into my new family. For that, I'm truly grateful. As a singer-song-writer and an ex-Navy SEAL/private military contractor, respectively, they could not be more diverse in their fields. However, both these guys are wicked smart and verbally adept in multiple areas of knowledge: science, religion, and physiology. In the beginning of our relationship, these guys became students of advanced metabolic function. They were as much a part of getting better as the advanced treatment protocols I developed. These guys can read blood work and steer people in the right direction when they can't get any answers from their physicians. Maybe this is why the three of us are so close; these guys didn't just talk the talk, they also walked the walk.

Ricky Zabala, ex-Special Forces, was the manager of Cigarz on the Avenue in Winter Park, Florida. I would see him occasionally and we would talk, both of us careful not to give up too much information. We trusted no one. We did this mental dance with each other many times. I could tell he was not going to talk about anything but the weather, my SWAT team background, and the fact that we had similar coping mechanisms. This gave Ricky the confidence that I was credible. Ricky was coming out of a dark place, and it was clear that he was working in the cigar store as a form of rehab, medicating his brain every day with simple carbohydrates and nicotine to keep his mood elevated. I couldn't push him; he had to move at his own pace. After about six months of sharing stories, Ricky started talking about his PTSD, which I related to immediately. He's an expert in dignitary protection, close-quarters combat, and small weapons, and worked undercover for the Orlando police. People in his line of work are constantly scanning the horizon for danger, even when there is no threat. This caused measurable physiological changes in his metabolism that his physicians did not understand. It's the kind of behavior he needed for survival in the war zone, but not in civilian life.

Ricky is a warrior with a unique skill set, but being hyperalert 24/7 causes a deficiency in the brain's feel-good neurotransmitter levels. This can lead to food, drug, or alcohol abuse. Ricky was consuming a high-carbohydrate diet, which was elevating his serotonin levels, keeping him in a good mood most of the time. He was close to 275 pounds with insulin resistance. It's extremely difficult to change a diet when a client has nutritional and hormonal deficiencies. The carbohydrates in his diet were likely the only thing keeping him sane. When a warrior has to integrate back into society, it makes no sense for the brain. When you are part of the "no-fuckin'-around crew," but now you have to go to Bed Bath & Beyond with your girlfriend or wife, it can be VERY surreal. People don't understand what war vets go through… and how could they? Most just care about what NFL games are on and whether or not they should splurge and get that new car.

Ricky had a strong belief in the traditional medical system. It became my job over the next few months to drip the science on him to open his mind and show him that our medical system is broken and that we are all getting bad information from our physicians. The good news was that Ricky was prescribed a handful of antidepressants and he refused to take them. This was an opportunity for me to build on. Many vets like Ricky can't shut their brains off, causing them to constantly cycle scenarios at night when they should be sleeping. The constant threat and situational awareness in the war zone changes the neurological architecture, which can lead to PTSD and depression. Ricky had friends who were emergency room physicians. I had to break it to him that these guys were no help to him. Just because you hear the word "doctor," don't assume that they can help you.

I walked Ricky through my plan, did some special blood tests not offered by conventional medicine, and we sat down with Sergio to do the evaluation. That was ground zero for Ricky's rehabilitation. Within six months of correcting his nutritional and hormonal deficiencies, as well as his diet, he lost fifty pounds of body fat and his mood improved exponentially. We formed an unbroken bond. I then moved on to help his family as well. His daughter was having difficulty conceiving a child, and we found out that she had very low progesterone, the hormone needed for the fetus to attach to the uterine wall. Once we corrected the deficiencies, she became pregnant. Ricky told me, "Every time I look at that baby, I think about you, Russ." His daughter-in-law had MS, and we developed a treatment protocol for that as well. Within a year, Ricky deeply believed in my skill set and wanted us to work together helping people. I asked Ricky to tell his story on my YouTube channel so we could help more war vets. He did the recording and it was amazing. Ricky's story was shot in one take, unedited, straight from the heart of someone who had been in the war zone, and the video resonated with thousands of people. The day I lost my folks, Ricky was right there beside me.

Erick Pace, lead singer of the godAmsterdams, spent many months in the hospital as a child with several infections of unknown origin. He was given high doses of Cipro (an antibiotic) for years, to the point where he could barely walk from the car to the physician's office fifty feet away. While spending time in the hospital alone, Erick found his passion for music. When I met Erick at my office, we went through the PowerPoint on the program. Shortly after that, we did some testing and found that he was extremely deficient on multiple metabolic levels. Erick was also under extreme stress. He was one of the owners of a dot-com that was being sold to a publicly traded company. At that time, he was in very poor health. We found that he had severe intestinal overgrowth. Remember, your intestinal flora helps you pull nutrients out of food. Due to his years of taking Cipro, he also had multiple nutritional and hormonal deficiencies. I had to turn this around for Erick, or his infections would come racing back. A healthy intestinal tract is critical for a strong immune system. I had to work fast to get Erick off those dangerous railroad tracks. He followed all my instructions and read the hundreds of e-mails I sent him. The best way to get well with any disease or illness is to do your own research and get a basic understanding of your condition while grasping the fact that your physician may not fully understand your condition. Erick quickly became a student of personalized medicine. Because of his unique skill set as a songwriter, we were always brainstorming on how to put complex medical terminology into a format that people could understand. Erick and I spent hours exchanging ideas. We knew that good content was the new oil. He was trying to get his songs into the public domain, while I was trying to do the same with my advanced treatment protocols, so we made a good team. In fact, we're still banging out ideas to this day.

Chapter Eleven

CARPE NOCTEM

The week after I found my folks, I didn't sleep. I was up for 96 hours straight and the stress was crushing me. I didn't have the endurance that I had in my twenties. I knew I was sliding into depression and I had to fix it immediately. Hacking my own brain was going to be a bitch. The visuals and anxiety of my past came rushing back, namely memories of all the bad shit I saw over the years. Those triggers never leave you. Traumatic events are imprinted in long-term storage. Evolutionary biologists say this is a survival tool passed down for millions of years, but I felt like it was killing me. I had to step it up, like I do for my clients, but now I had to do it for myself.

I had my doctor run lab work so I could adjust my hormone levels with a focus on the feel-good neurotransmitters serotonin and dopamine. It was important for me to stay busy. As soon as I had any dead air, I would get a flashing image of the position in which I found my mother and father... their clothes and jewelry... even their facial expressions... in vivid detail. I was gut punched. I kept thinking, *What were my last words to them?* I tried hard to remember. I wanted to slow down and deconstruct the very last time we spent together. I needed to remember our good times. Was this healthy? I'm not sure, but it was cycling through my mind every few minutes. It was so sudden, finding them... I just went over to their house to say hello and was hit in the face with a tragic bat. I didn't get a chance to say goodbye or "I love you, Mom. I love you, Dad." *Nothing.* These thoughts kept cycling in my head.

To the people who told me God was looking out for me, I said, "Fuck God! If He let this happen versus having my parents pass one at a time, then God's an illusion, like Santa and the fucking Easter Bunny." Even as an altar boy in one of the largest Catholic churches in New Jersey, I didn't buy into the God bullshit. It was just one more social control mechanism. *People are born into original sin...* Please!

Writing these lines is what's saving my life, particularly remembering my mother, who had an amazing sense of humor. She was that person who made everyone feel comfortable, one of the few people who made me laugh—hard. She was also tough as hell. My father was a union leader in Jersey, and that life took a special woman. My mother and father were the classic story of *opposites attract.* My old man was intense and passionate. He never told me he loved me or handed out compliments; he just got me ready for the ass kicking life would hand out. He did what he thought was best, but I must say, when my father turned 85 years old, he let me take him to my physician for testosterone and thyroid hormone, as he was deficient in both. Once we corrected his hormonal levels, he cut his insulin dose in half. Insulin is not a cure for diabetes; it's the cause. Insulin damages multiple systems and can lead to blindness, heart disease, and amputations. That is how toxic insulin is for the body. I watched my father struggle with diabetes, but he never worried about dieting... it was always a fear of blindness. He was fearful of insulin, as it causes the small arteries in the eyes to burst, so the protocol I developed for my father was intended to stabilize his illness. One day, out of the blue, my father called me. He never called me, so I initially thought it was an emergency, that something had happened to my mother. I answered the call and he said, "Russ, I have to thank you," words I'd never heard.

I said, "What's up, Dad?"

He said, "I'm sitting here with an erection… so I want to say thanks."

I laughed and said, "That's a good sign, Dad. The blood to your brain and heart will improve too."

He said, "That's good, so I'll be smarter too." Then he said, "I'll see ya later," and hung up.

He was always brief in his conversations with me. I know that he was a good man struggling with a devastating illness. If testosterone helped the circulation to his penis, then it would definitely help the blood circulation to his eyes. The conventional treatment for diabetes is wrong—completely wrong—but that's all changing as I write these lines.

When I was out all night with girls, my mother would ask, "Where were you?"

I always said, "Church, Mom. I went to church."

Her response was always, "You're pulling my leg, Russ. I know where you were."

She lived for the church and went to mass three times a week. I loved to joke about all that praying she was doing, and my mother would just laugh and roll with it. If it made her feel good, then who was I to say otherwise?

I got into trouble when I was a kid a few times and was taken to the police station. She would have to come get me, so as I joked with her, she would say, "Hey! You'd still be in jail if it wasn't for me, kiddo." Mom almost passed out when I first told her that I was going to the police academy.

My father used words that made me think when I got in trouble: "You're embarrassing the family! Christ, what's wrong with you? Your mother had three miscarriages before you came along… don't be the fourth."

Funny enough, it's those times I'm trying so desperately to hang on to.

I needed sleep. Man, if I could just pass out for an hour, just to turn my brain off. Maybe this was the night… For the past year, I had been working on developing a program using lucid dreaming for war vets, so I applied many of the concepts to myself. Lucid dreaming is where you can take control of your dreams. It is a skill that must be practiced every day. While in the dream, you have to look for cues. The one I notice that tells me I'm jacked into the dream state is when I pass by a mirror in a lucid dream. The reflection is not me; it's someone else. This cue allows me to start to control the dream, allowing me to run, fly, jump over buildings… anything is possible. Lucid dreaming is as strong as any drug and just like a drug; when I woke up, I wanted more. This type of dream state was truly an experience I'd never before felt in my life, but the trick is to take control, rather than be a passenger. That is the part that takes time to master. While lucid dreaming, you can talk to people and see their faces. It's all in color… the buildings, the cars on the street… it's like another world. I've done it five times, but can't repeat it on demand. I never know when it's coming, so I just maintain my same routine. I experiment with nootropics: lithium, nicotine, GABA, and 5HTP to help me jump off into the lucid dreaming state. At times, I couldn't tell the difference between reality and lucid dreaming. It seems *that* real. I thought it could be a powerful tool to help heal people after traumatic situations. I hypothesized that if you can take control of the situation in your dream, it could be healing by providing closure. No more endless "coulda, woulda, shoulda" thoughts. You could end the constant scenarios going through your head and wake up cleansed.

It had only been five days, but the lack of sleep was elevating my cortisol (stress hormone) level. My dosing all had to change as I stabilized my brain chemistry and neurotransmitter levels. I was going to take a deep dive into the dream state. I was in nutritional ketosis (fat burning) and had to switch to a high-carbohydrate diet at night just to get that burst of serotonin that would calm my brain chemistry and help it stop cycling thoughts. Pasta, white rice, and bread became my go-to food for a few days. The book *Potatoes Not Prozac* by Dr. Kathleen DesMaisons speaks to the research of using carbohydrates to manipulate brain chemistry.

My clients started to notice that something was wrong. I would drift off in our conversation and they knew it. These clients were paying the bills, but I was slipping. I had to boost my focus before things got any worse. I'd used carbohydrates with addicts in the past and began to feel the effects. After dinner around 7:00, I would get a blast of glucose circulating in my bloodstream. If I was watching TV and started feeling sleepy, I would immediately get up and go to bed, lie on my back, and wait until everything went dark. The next morning, it would feel like I had a hangover because the elevated insulin had caused fluid retention. When I checked my blood glucose, it would be about 160. I thought, *Great, I'm on my way to diabetes.* I also knew that my blood glucose had to be under 100 to hit the lucid dreaming state in the morning.

As my eyes would slowly open and I would realize that I was awake, my very first thought would shoot like a lightning bolt to my mother and father. I could not remember my last conversation with them. *What had we talked about?* I wanted to relive that time so desperately. I've worked with people in traumatic situations who cycled the same thoughts over and over, so I understood what I had to do. Taking the time to write this book allowed me to focus and shut my brain off for a few hours a day. Anger was working inside of me like an organ, secreting pain and anxiety, and I was becoming a different person. Fortunately, one of my skills is to hyperfocus, which allowed me to exhale and start the healing process.

For years, responding to emergency calls and racing long distances caused elevations in cortisol, which splashed off my hippocampus, damaging my short-term memory. All incoming data has to be processed at the hippocampus tollbooth before moving on to long-term storage. No matter where I was in Winter Park, I would lose my car and forget where I parked it. Feeling these unusual effects scared me into taking more action. I started fasting, only eating one meal in 24 hours. This allowed my brain to burn a ketone called BHB for fuel, rather than glucose. This also raised my levels of another feel-good neurotransmitter called GABA. I would run, but I kept my heart rate down, nothing intense and never over three miles or thirty minutes, just enough to boost my mood.

My physicians addressed my testosterone, thyroid, and adrenal deficiencies, which I felt within 24 hours. That was good. Testosterone elevates dopamine levels when combined with aerobic exercise. Brain-derived neurotropic factor increases as well, but not many physicians know this. Brain-derived neurotropic factor stimulates neurogenesis, the manufacture of new cells. New cells not compromised by cortisol. Remember, among other effects, excess cortisol damages short-term memory. I remained focused on my clients, which allowed me to feel productive and focus my mind on helping people using my unique skill set.

The sense of self-worth helped me power through the trauma of losing my parents and feeling alone for the first time in my life. It also helped that I knew I had done right by them. I'd had my mother and father on the advanced treatment protocols and they had been doing fantastic. After all they had done for me, I had been able to improve their quality of life, which made me feel good.

I was the go-to guy. I was the guy who helped people through the worst times in their lives. Now, few were here for me. People would contact me on Facebook or come up to me on the street, but these people just wanted details of what happened. I had no interest in reliving the scene in my head. I was given the gift of reading people early on in life. Maybe it evolved from coming face-to-face with so many sick people, talking to them and holding their hands. This taught me an incredible amount about human nature. Most of the people who I encountered that week were basically worthless. They saw me all the time, but now they were suddenly concerned. Please! They all saw the police and emergency vehicles in front of my parents' home. They just wanted details, not to offer any real help.

Like any trauma in life, the only way around is to go straight through it, and I knew that I would eventually overcome my loss. I was starting to sleep better, and I was able to back off the carbohydrates around day nine. I was starting to crack into the dream state and could see certain images, but would wake up every few hours, walk around the house, and then go back to bed for another try. You have to get up multiple times a night—every 3 to 4 hours—to stimulate lucid dreaming.

There's something critical about breaking up the sleep intervals. The first time I ever entered a lucid dream, there was no beginning and no ending. I was just there. I was in a large medical rehab center for war vets. I walked from bed to bed talking to the vets and looking at their injuries, even noting the detail of surgical pins inserted into a femur... the long bone in the leg was amazingly detailed. I saw broken legs in traction and lacerations. All the patients were awake and in a good mood while talking to me. I remember their faces, the hospital grounds, what they wore...everything. I knew I could take control of the dream when a physician walked up to me wearing a white lab coat over his suit, but he was also wearing a blue baseball cap. No logos, just blue. This was an obvious clue. I reached out and took the cap off his head, looked at it, and then placed it back on his head. At that point, I knew I was lucid dreaming. When I woke up, I couldn't wait to go back, and I kept trying for the next three weeks, but to no avail. I was always worried about the dream taking a turn and returning to my traumatic memories, but so far, all the dreams had been pleasant. Nonetheless, I was still cautious.

I increased my meds, a combination that was customized for my current sleep deprivation that included GABA, 5HTP, transdermal progesterone, and low-dose lithium. I really needed this brain hack to work. I just hoped that the planets would align so I could sleep through one night. The progesterone, when it metabolized, had an amazing narcotic effect. I would rub it on my skin at night and it would elevate brain neurotransmitters. Progesterone binds to the same brain receptor sites as Prozac and Xanax, and is also much safer to use. I cut the carbohydrates completely out of my diet and went back into ketosis. I kept hoping that something would happen. Many people who have experienced traumatic events never fully recover, a fact that was in the back of my mind as well.

The fact that my mother and father were dead, that I would never see or talk to them again, was very hard to wrap my head around. I was still dazed and was trying to focus my thoughts, so I could be strong for my sister. Kathy was extremely close to my parents, and their death hit her hard. I had been around dying people most of my life, but Kathy hadn't. I didn't want her to know the details. It would be too hard for her to deal with. She was all the family I had left and I wanted to keep her healthy.

The next morning, I woke up after another night of no dreaming. I was a little groggy, so I decreased my dose of GABA. When you take too much GABA, it can make you feel extremely fatigued. The phone rang and it was my buddy, Scott Levitt. As I mentioned previously, Scott was an extremely gifted cyclist and endurance athlete. It had been ten years since he'd had his heart attack, which had precipitated the battle we fought with his cardiologists, who had no idea how to take care of an athlete like him.

Scott told me that our mutual friend, Mick Night, was in a bad place. Mick and I had been friends for years. A few days earlier, Mick's son, John Michael, had had pain in the back of his head and Mick had driven him to the hospital. The pain intensified, and an artery burst in John Michael's brain stem, causing complete paralysis. It's called locked-in syndrome. The movie *The Diving Bell and the Butterfly* was about this condition. When Scott finished the story, I said, "Scott, let me dive into this. I've got all the newest research on stroke recovery."

When Scott hung up, I went on a sixteen-hour research marathon. I called Chrissy, one of my writers, and told her that I would be sending research reports all night, and asked her to arrange them and put them in a file. Chrissy is one of the few people on the planet who understands the way I work. As patterns connect and the screens drop down in my brain, I have to utilize stream-of-consciousness writing, just letting thoughts flow from my head to my fingers. I've written for six hours before just using a cellphone keyboard. After these sessions, I have to shut my brain off to quiet the constant thoughts. I usually just go to a movie—any movie—and try to escape for a bit. This allows my prefrontal cortex, where all executive thinking takes place, to quiet down. The dark, cool movie theater provides a calming environment for my brain. I've learned skills from high-level code writers and Special Forces personnel that I regularly apply to my behavior. I would not consume anything but black coffee when I needed to focus, which has a paradoxical effect on me. Caffeine calms me down. Like any person suffering from ADHD or dyslexia, I had to find my own ways over the years to deal with distraction and lack of focus. I used to try to explain this to people; I've learned it's better to just keep it to myself.

I desperately wanted to help John Michael. The brain rehab data I collected on Louis Amabile and the treatment I had designed for his recovery would be a big part, along with the notes I took when neurologists Dr. Ira Goodman and Dr. Arnaldo Isa took the time to talk to me a few years ago during my research. Now, fMRI advanced imaging allows neuroradiologists to see inside the brain on a cellular level in real time. This imaging was changing the treatment strategy for strokes and brain injuries.

John Michael was undergoing stroke rehabilitation at the Shepherd Center in Atlanta, one of the best in the country. First, we had to examine all its protocols, along with the Mayo Clinic's treatment plan. My team and I planned to develop a visual and graphic presentation that Mick Night would understand, as well as the physicians. In situations like this, the family is told many things and it gets confusing. We didn't want to add to the confusion.

Thoughts of my mother and father disappeared during my intervals of extreme concentration as I pulled the research together. I noticed this early on, so I developed another part of the treatment plan each day. I maintained my medication regimen each night with the hopes of achieving extended REM sleep the next morning. I did a finger stick to check my blood glucose with a ketone blood monitor. I was still in nutritional ketosis. I felt energized and excited. One day, I met Trent and Chrissy at the film studio to storyboard the protocol we were developing for John Michael because it never had been done before, and we wanted the family to understand it. After we storyboarded the video at the studio, I headed home. I didn't even take my clothes off, just fell into bed and went to sleep. And that's when it happened.

I used my key to unlock the door of my parents' home. Once inside, I walked back to my mother's room, where she had the TV on. When she saw me, she smiled and said, "Son, come here and sit down." She patted the end of the bed. I couldn't believe what I was seeing. I blurted out, "Mom! I thought you died. I checked you."

She said, "Are you crazy? Christ, and you were a paramedic."

I said, "Mom, I checked you myself; I thought you were dead."

Again, she smiled and said, "No, son, I'm right here," and she held both my hands.

I could feel the veins underneath her fair Irish skin and traced them to her wrists, where they disappeared under the sleeves of her blue dress. I held my breath. I questioned whether I had made a mistake. Adrenaline pumped through my body. I was so truly and deeply happy to see my mother; talking to her gave me such relief. It allowed me to exhale for the first time since finding her. My mom's smile and her blue eyes had such clarity, something I'd never seen in anyone else. I kept holding her hands. I didn't want to let go. I had the fear that I would lose her again. That's when my mom said, "Come, let's go get something to eat."

With a sigh of relief, I said, "Okay," even though I wasn't hungry. I was just so excited to see her. As I got up from my mom's bed and turned to the chest of drawers, I walked past the mirror and stopped on a dime. My stomach dropped and the sadness rose up; the reflection was not me.

I'd had none of the cues of going into a lucid dream, so when I saw my mother, it had felt incredibly real. Just being able see my mom and talk to her was healing. I got to hold her hand, look into her eyes, and laugh with her one more time. I wanted to repeat everything I had done the day before—eat the same food and take the same meds in the same order. I wanted to try for a talk with my father next.

I didn't let that distract me from the work we were doing for John Michael, though. After completing advanced testing on him, we uncovered metabolic deficiencies not found at the Shepherd Center. He is a brave young man and is still fighting for recovery.

Chapter Twelve

CHASING THE DRAGON

I hit the on-ramp of Interstate 4 at 80 MPH, took a long pull off a Marlboro Red, and held it deep in my lungs. The nicotine would cross my blood-brain barrier in eight seconds, allowing me to relax and hyperfocus on the highway ahead. I gripped the steering wheel at ten and two. I was driving to save a friend, and all I could think about was that she was in respiratory arrest. The one person I truly cared about was going to die if I didn't get to her. My brain and reflexes auto-loaded skills I'd learned while responding to fire calls. A truck carrying 2,000 gallons of water doesn't stop when you hit the brakes, so I had to anticipate 500 yards ahead on every emergency response. My reaction time has always been insanely fast, and in that moment, a lifetime of skills was focused on getting to Michelle.

If her brain was starved of oxygen for more than four minutes, brain damage and respiratory arrest would set in. Or, if she vomited and tried to take a breath, she could aspirate and die of suffocation, just like so many college students who get wasted on drinking games their freshman year.

I punched the gas pedal and kicked it up to 100 MPH, weaving in and out of vehicles frozen at the speed limit. Despite the high speed and my concern for Michelle, my pulse rate remained low. My foot slid off the gas pedal and expertly tapped the brakes. I was dialed in, just like old times. I was not going to have another friend die, no fucking way!

When I'd gotten the call from Michelle, she could barely speak, slurring her words, trying to gather her thoughts and not forming complete sentences. Her voice, pitch, tone, and cadence were all off. The meds were taking over her brain.

I said, "Michelle, come on, baby, focus. Tell me where you are… come on!"

She would answer with a "Yes" and then drift off to another conversation.

"Michelle, where are you, baby? Talk to me. Jesus Christ!"

I knew instantly that this was bad, and then I heard someone in the background say, "Arnold Palmer." It clicked. I ran out the door and jumped into my car.

She had made it to the hospital waiting room at Arnold Palmer Hospital. That's what I'm talking about. Michelle knew, as she felt the medication take over, to walk in the direction of the hospital.

I had a destination, but I was still fifteen miles away. I knew that the idiots at the rehab center had her on a dangerous combination of methadone, antidepressant, and who knows what else. She weighed a little over a hundred pounds, so it didn't take much to suppress her respiration and heart rate. These methadone clinics overprescribe and kill people all the time. A year prior, a physician prescribed oxycodone to Michelle for back pain. She quickly became addicted. When the script ran out, withdrawals hit her like a sucker punch to the face. When she called her physicians, they could offer no help.

For those who don't know, withdrawals are emotionally, mentally, and physically painful. Even a blanket on a person's skin can cause pain. Michelle's only available option was heroin, which allowed her to feel normal and get through the day. Opiate addiction is not about getting high, but rather about feeling normal. Fortunately, she kicked the heroin habit and was taking methadone to stay clean, but methadone is still an opiate. Combine the methadone with alcohol and an addict can often find peace.

This was the completely wrong treatment protocol for Michelle, but when her family got involved, I had to step away, even though it was painful to watch. I even took the new research over to her family, but they did nothing. I was also consulting with the New Bridge Addiction Center at the time, but no one would listen. Michelle's life had been flipped upside down when the father of her five-year-old daughter had died. I remember the day she called me; she was absolutely heartbroken. My executive assistant found Michelle crying a few times in our office break room; her stress was clearly becoming overwhelming.

Michelle cares deeply about people and has never met a stranger. It isn't a façade either. Working with me was her passion, but she was questioned about it daily by her mother, who was a midwife, and her father, who was a pharmacist. She would come home and share the new research she was learning, and they would take turns trying to discredit what she was sharing. The good news was that by going toe-to-toe with her mom and dad, Michelle was gaining an important skill set. I knew that if we got through those early days, she would be an excellent intervention specialist with my team. I meet very few people in life who are just good people, like it was hardwired in their DNA. Michelle is one of these rare individuals. She didn't have the skills to get better, but she desperately wanted to get these drugs out of her system for her daughter's sake.

You may have a picture in your mind of what an addict looks like, but it's probably wrong. I know moms, dads, priests, police officers, physicians, teachers, and high-level executives who are addicts. I never judged; I just helped them get well. Family members don't have the skills or the training to take care of someone they love who is addicted, so the yelling and fighting starts. Michelle called me one time and said, "I'm a bad mom."

I replied, "You're trying to get over an illness that your family doesn't understand. It's like getting mad at a diabetic for taking insulin."

Thoughts of Michelle and our history were bouncing around in my head, swinging between memories of the good and painful times.

I was five miles away, still flying down Interstate 4, pumping the brakes and weaving around cars, before moving to the right-hand lane to exit the highway. Arnold Palmer Hospital was a block from the interstate, but police were everywhere, so I had to pull back on the speed. I finally made it and pulled up to the entrance of the hospital. I parked and threw the valet my keys before bolting inside to the waiting room. Scanning the rows of people, I found Michelle sitting with her head completely back, mouth wide open, snoring. When I saw her take a breath, I knew we were good. I slowly walked over to keep people from staring. I placed the palm of my hand on the back of her head and gently moved it to an upright position.

"Michelle." I shook her, and then shook her again. She opened those baby blues and smiled. "You scared the shit out of me, buddy."

Michelle was looking around and gathering her thoughts, undoubtedly wondering how she had gotten to the hospital waiting room. "Michelle. What happened?"

I already knew. The dose of methadone was too high and it had interacted with the antidepressants.

I could see that Michelle was sweating, pale, and hypoglycemic. I said, "Can you stand?" I helped her get to her feet. "Come on, let's go."

Michelle got up and walked over to the vending machine. Staring down at the selection, she looked at me and said, "Which snack is low carb?"

I laughed. "You're fucking kidding me, right? You have how many drugs in your system? Christ, just get a Snickers bar." I was just so grateful to see her standing, alive and talking, and she was worried about her weight.

"Michelle, the Snickers will bump up your blood glucose fast." Snickers bar in hand, Michelle and I walked to the car. A false alarm. She hadn't died. She hadn't suffocated in her own vomit. She was okay.

Looking at her walking to the car, I was thinking that I had helped cancer patients achieve remission and had developed advanced brain rehab programs, but addictions… that was a different evil that stole the souls of good people. I knew how to beat it, but getting the addiction specialists to sign off was always a problem. Those arrogant assholes just couldn't believe it when I put the research into their hands and said, "Let's pull the trigger on this, Doc, and you'll be a rock star giving lectures around the world by next year."

I tried to navigate Michelle away from all the slick AA experts who think it's their way or the highway. I was on the phone with one of these assholes who tried to get in the way of Michelle's intervention. He called me chaotic, so I called him a weak genetic mutation. Michelle, due to her low neurotransmitter levels, thought the sun rose and set on this idiot.

It was just a few years ago that the advanced imaging of the brain called fMRI first allowed us to see that the brain continues to grow until we die. This is called neurogenesis. Many physicians don't understand that opiates can stimulate neurogenesis, meaning that the addiction becomes hardwired into living brain tissue. This is called opiate-induced neuroplasticity. This knowledge will change current addiction treatment.

At one point, my team was invited to the grand opening of an addiction center. These places are cash cows, but they're not really practicing good scientific research. It's all about the money, to the tune of $10,000–$15,000 for seven days, but what goes on in those seven to ten days isn't very impressive. Addiction is so rampant that centers have popped up like weeds all over Florida. Just study the history. We are a drug-taking species; in 1903, Coca-Cola was manufactured as an intellect-stimulating beverage that contained 60 mg of cocaine per 8 ounces.

I decided to keep my mouth shut during the meeting with the owners of the center; I knew that the program we developed could change the way addicts get treated, but would they buy into it?

My research into the metabolic deficiencies caused by addictions started when I met the owners of RX Development, Tom Mollick and Marty Krytus, in 2009. Their medication dispensing company is in thirteen states and there are 700 pain management physicians connected to their program. Both owners are on my program and are good friends. I've met many of the pain management physicians and drilled down with them on the nutritional and hormonal deficiencies caused by a wide variety of pain medications. I developed testing and treatment protocols to upregulate the metabolism after using pain meds, allowing these people to get back to life and quit being the walking dead. I wanted to make a difference and pull the trigger, but

God, do things move slowly. Meeting after meeting, physicians were data mining my program, and many of the executives were simply trying to figure out how the hell I came up with this. More importantly, they wanted to lock me into some exclusivity contract. Fortunately, I always had the upper hand because I didn't give a shit about the money. If they didn't buy into the idea, I would just open source it.

The intestinal tract is now considered a secondary brain, and if the beneficial flora in the gut fall out of balance, it will affect brain chemistry. Research exists on what is called the opiate bowel, namely how opiates can damage the intestinal tract. This research is all new, by the way. That being said, we have to go slow, because even certified physicians who are considered addiction specialists are COMPLETELY LOST when it comes to advanced treatment that tests multiple nutritional and hormonal deficiencies that can help an addict recover. I would sit right across from these guys explaining the new research, and they would shake their heads, denying that it could possibly work.

I've been to addiction centers that charge $20,000–$40,000 a month and all they do is talk therapy. However, with the multiple layers of complexity in the brain, the intestinal tract connection, and opiates causing damage on the cellular level, addiction has to be reversed with nutritional and hormonal support, not feel-good conversation.

I've worked with people addicted to alcohol, heroin, methadone, carbohydrates, and exercise, among other things. Every case came down to understanding brain chemistry. There are approximately 86 billion neurons with 100 trillion connections inside our head. These numbers are admittedly hard to wrap your head around. The important thing to know is that each addict is biochemically unique, meaning that one treatment protocol won't work for everyone. I will make one sweeping generalization: testing for and correcting multiple nutritional and hormonal deficiencies is a basic protocol that can be applied to everyone.

Rehab facilities are growing by the tens of thousands across the United States. Keeping up with the demand, many are just taking insurance money, and families drain their bank accounts because they want their child back, healthy and happy. Each facility uses slick marketing, with pictures of the beach as a hook. In the end, the people that go through these programs frequently relapse, because drugs hardwire the brain for negative behaviors. It takes years to reprogram an addict; it's difficult, but it can be done.

Someone doesn't just wake up one morning and say, "Today, I think I'll do heroin." It's a multifactorial process. Getting these people better takes a lot more than talk therapy; we have to treat multiple metabolic systems. The dopamine burst you get from heroin is mind-boggling. Let me explain. On a scale of 1 to 1000, eating a bagel may bump you to 50, a shot of testosterone is 150, and an orgasm tops out around 200. The first shot of heroin rings the bell at 800, so it's easy to see why it's so addicting for some people after a single high. After each hit, they'll need a larger dose to experience the same effect. Chasing the dragon becomes a way of life. The emotional and intellectual capital that goes into deprograming these kids can make you sick if you're not fit. If you want to do high-level interventions, you need to be in shape. This is not a sprint, it's a marathon… and detox is mile one.

Addicts are just regular people trying to feel normal. Most addicts I work with need a bump every four hours at $20 to $30 a shot. Many addicts are spending $1,800 to $2,000 a month just to get through the day and feel normal. The dealers in my area, which is a college town, have an average of 200 to 500 clients, so do the math. The bling-bling factor is very real. These devils in plain clothes are rockin' the lifestyle. Thankfully, some of my clients are PMC (Private Military Contract) from what used to be called Blackwater. I need men with that special skill set to watch my back.

My connections from when I was on the SWAT team were also very helpful, but I was never strapped in meetings with dealers. I just talked straight and paid them off to stay away from my clients—end of story.

My drug box and telemetry radio saved lives back when I was a paramedic, but my toolbox had to change. When I needed to detox a 25-year-old who had been using heroin for two years, I attacked the problem with a different set of tools, consisting of intravenous antioxidants, followed by daily injections of nutritional and hormonal support, which would help rebuild the mitochondria on a cellular level. The mitochondria power every cell in the body to make ATP, which is basically energy.

An addict's diet has to change if he or she wants to get healthy. Fasting and a ketogenic (fat-burning) diet are helpful, as they activate brain-derived neurotropic factor, which is basically Miracle-Gro for the brain. During the detox process, these folks have extremely intense cravings for sugar and carbohydrates. Sugar and carbohydrates elevate levels of the feel-good neurotransmitter, serotonin. There's a reason diabetes is such a problem with younger and younger people. Sugar, and simple carbs that easily turn into sugar, are addictive. There's plenty of documentation and books on the subject.

The reason AA only has a twenty-five percent success rate is that alcohol is basically a super carbohydrate. During an AA meeting, look at the back table. It's like Halloween—candy and carbs everywhere. Even when alcoholics aren't drinking, they're still hitting the same brain receptors with massive carb intakes. In my experience with addicts, alcohol is actually much harder to quit than heroin.

Another crucial part of the detox process is that the client must be ready to step up. By that point, many of them have already burned every bridge and stolen from family members. Everyone in their life has basically thrown their hands in the air. However, these are not bad people. They have a disease, but you don't go to jail for diabetes, so I get it.

There are multiple layers of complexity to the metabolism during this treatment, so given my competitive nature, I, Russ Scala, go to battle with the addiction. I know this is my calling, which is probably why I'm still single. I'm focused, obsessed, and I don't sleep for days while I'm plugged in to a challenge. I'm still doing what I did in the eighties. I save lives.

Chapter Thirteen

WHY WE BELIEVE

The third leading cause of death in the US is our own medical system. Hard to believe, isn't it? These are called iatrogenic deaths—deaths caused by the healer. A recent Johns Hopkins study has determined that over 250,000 deaths stem from medical errors per year, which puts it third behind heart disease and cancer, respectively.[1] Some estimates for iatrogenic death are higher. The *Journal of Patient Safety* states between 210,000 and 440,000 patients each year go to the hospital and suffer some type of preventable harm that contributes to their death.[2] "Properly" prescribed drugs (not counting misprescribed or misused drugs) cause 1.9 million hospitalizations a year. A 2011 review of hospital charts reported that adverse drug reactions caused 2.1 million injuries in the US and 128,000 deaths in a year's time.

1 McMains, Vanessa. "Johns Hopkins study suggests medical errors are third-leading cause of death in U.S." hub.jhu.edu. https://hub.jhu.edu/2016/05/03/medical-errors-third-leading-cause-of-death/

2 Allen, Marshall. "How Many Die From Medical Mistakes In U.S. Hospitals?" NPR.org. http://www.npr.org/sections/health-shots/2013/09/20/224507654/how-many-die-from-medical-mistakes-in-u-s-hospitals

The number of people exposed to unnecessary hospitalization is 8.9 million.[3]

The perception that the US has the highest quality of medical care in the world is blatantly false. The American healthcare system currently ranks 37th in the world, as stated by the World Health Organization.[4] I get a pain in the pit of my stomach when I think of good people being taken by the hand, told that everything is going to be fine, and then ending up severely damaged or dead. People can only fight this by changing what they believe, asking the tough questions, and getting educated in basic biology. Medical tourism outside the US is a billion-dollar business that reflects this growing trend.

How do we get people to change their belief systems, and thus their behavior, when billions are spent on advertising every year for drugs and treatments that don't work? These stats are as sad as they are scary. Just think about the long list of side-effect disclaimers that finish off every TV drug commercial.

I basically have to create a social media SWAT team to drip the science on people. As you read these lines, the treatments for heart disease, diabetes, obesity, cancer, and mental illness are changing. Soon, there will be no more monotherapy (one drug for one disease). Billions will be lost by conventional medicine and billions more will be made by the innovative early adaptors who develop the next great

3   Light, Donald. "New Prescription Drugs: A Major Health Risk With Few Offsetting Advantages." ethics.harvard.edu. http://ethics.harvard.edu/blog/new-prescription-drugs-major-health-risk-few-offsetting-advantages

4   "World Health Organization's Ranking of the World's Health Systems." ThePatientFactor.com. http://thepatientfactor.com/canadian-health-care-information/world-health-organizations-ranking-of-the-worlds-health-systems/

business models. This will not come from large institutions; it will come from people like you reading this book. There are already groups of regular people on Facebook saving lives every day by sharing their stories. Many of these folks have tens of thousands of followers. This evolution of thought is happening now. Creating the best content to educate people will be the next paradigm.

Before I get into how my team of five people—a singer-songwriter, a horror movie director, a writer, a single mom, and me—are going to change medicine forever using our collective skill set and social media, let's first start with a bit of history about my belief systems. What was my motivation to change my behaviors and what got me out of bed every morning to roll the boulder back up the hill?

As a child, I was taught not to interrupt and to listen to the adults. The thing is, I had questions—a lot of them. Also, sprinkle in a little ADHD and dyslexia. Basically, I was a pain in the ass to adults. I would hear the phrase, "Christ, you again? What do you want now?" I was the same way when I had the run of the hospital, asking questions on every floor, from the ER to CCU. I noticed the hypocrisy early on with priests, nuns, lay teachers, police, and my patients' conflicting belief systems on the same subjects. Life. Listening to what and why people believe in certain subject matters made me think about where they got their information. Books, Bibles, or Bullshit were the three Bs of manufacturing an enemy. The Devil, global warming, Communism, power, political gain, or now—the biggie—terrorism. To get a consensus across the board and change thinking, we need a boogieman.

I ask myself in every situation, *How do I get to the core of this issue? How can I find the answers fast and change people's thinking with simple statements, something like 'Fat is critical for the brain and cells to function?* For 50 years, millions of people were convinced that fat causes heart attacks and should therefore not be part of the human diet, or should at least be vilified and highly controlled. The idea that fat is bad is a belief system perpetuated by mainstream media and the AMA, so people became convinced fat was dangerous. This thinking was totally wrong. I mean, the lipid bilayer of trillions of cells is composed of fat. Our brains are made of fats. How they convinced the public that fat was bad is just an amazing marketing campaign that worked brilliantly.

As a kid, I was mesmerized by the church, which uses the same social control mechanisms as conventional medicine. So, I had to think back, *What changed my belief system then?* If you think about it, you have a book, repetitive training, and a community that believes and meets on a regular basis. This is how minds are altered in one specific direction. *So... how do I put a dent in this armor?* As I mentioned, my friend, Erick Pace, is a songwriter for the godAmsterdams. He took me to his recording studio and taught me about everything that went into making a song, namely the multiple layers of complexity to master a song until it is radio ready. I have never listened to music the same way because Erick took the time to educate me and show me the steps. As you can imagine, my brain lit up like a Christmas tree. Erick taught people with songs and I needed a similar skill set. What makes a person repeat the same words while tapping their foot to the beat? I knew that this was big. Listening to the priests at mass and then listening to people's interpretations of those words was always interesting. That sermon meant different things to different people, yet they had all heard the same song. I continued to wrack my brain, thinking back to those defining moments in my life that had changed my belief system.

The Catholic school I went to was heavy on the indoctrination process. I could not articulate what it was in my nine-year-old mind, but my gut told me this was all just made up. My beautiful Irish Catholic mother was so proud of me when I became an altar boy and served my first mass. I remember her taking pictures of me while I was holding the chalice for the priest. I looked out at the congregation from the altar and my mom was in the first row with a huge smile on her face.

I had to study Latin, and repeat the words back as a test in front of the Gestapo-like nuns. The first time Sister Mary cracked me in the face with the open palm of her hand for talking in church, I kicked her in the leg and got sent home. My mother was thunderstruck. My father said "Good" and told my mother, "No one touches my fucking kids." Then he looked at me. "Don't you ever take any shit from anybody!" He followed that with, "Listen to me, okay? Listen! I want you to stay away from Father Dailey and Father Cook, you hear me? And if you're alone with them, you tell me everything they say to you." My old man knew what he was talking about and thank God for that, because abuse was rampant in our church. I remember the priests being driven around in black limos. The adult married women would just swoon while talking to the priests after mass. These guys were like celebrities, which I never understood. As a kid, I was already onto their bullshit behavior. They were sly, but so was I. *I'm doing the work of God"* was a phrase I would always hear. I remember getting told to sit down and shut up, and that I was going to hell for asking so many questions. Decoding the adult language of religion was confusing for me. At that time, I only thought there was one religion—Catholic, that was it. I had no idea that others existed. Yep, I was drinking the Kool-Aid pretty early.

Imagine that, three persons in one God? Really? How does that work? Babies are born into sin? Babies? What did they do? So, Purgatory is a place to burn off sins, and then you can enter Heaven after spending a day or two there? A celestial timeout for players to be named later? But if a baby dies before being baptized, it will forever be in Limbo? What the fuck is Limbo? What a shame for parents to think that if they happen to lose a baby. My mother had three miscarriages and that always affected her. People give Scientology a hard time; I see no difference.

This confusion at such a young age just caused me to question more institutions, from religion to healthcare. I've always asked questions and never thought that I knew it all. Every time I finished a book, hundreds of doors and questions would open up in my mind. I would constantly run scenarios in my head, obsessing over what was going on internally with people. Listening is critical for my work. From triathletes and heroin addicts to celebrities and single moms and dads, their stories have always guided me in drilling down on an intervention. Listening and immersing myself in different cultures truly showed me the meaning and intention behind the thoughts and actions of people: the police officer who beat the shit out of a drunk driver for no reason, the executive getting busted for insider trading with a keystroke, a mother with post-partum depression that drowns her baby for crying... Again, I was never quick with answers, but listening gave me a road map of the behavioral dominoes that had fallen to make them think this way and justify their bat-shit-crazy behavior.

As a child, I viewed every adult as wearing a mask, meaning that the person I was meeting may not be the real person. My father was a big part of that educational process. When I made stupid mistakes, I would've welcomed a beating from him. A few minutes of pain and it would be over, but he was too slick. My father knew what I needed. When his family dog had too many puppies that they couldn't afford to feed, it was my dad's job at ten years of age to go down to the waterfront and drown the puppies. He left home at 16 in the 1940s to become a merchant marine sailor and traveled the world before he was 20. Hard times make hard people. My father was trying in his own way to get me ready for the hardest knocks of life, making sure I didn't just curl up on the floor when shit happened. When I hit a neighbor in the eye with a rock, my father didn't beat me; he made me wear a blindfold. I never picked up a rock again. When I came home drunk after stealing a bottle of whiskey from a friend's home, he didn't yell at me; he put me in the car and drove me down to the local bar, took me inside, and pointed to the people at the bar. "Keep drinking, Russ, and you will end up like these fucking losers. You wanna end up like that?" When my father caught me and my girlfriend in my room messing around, he said, "Think what would happen if someone was doing that with your sister? What if you got that girl pregnant? Think about all those assholes in your school that would call her a whore. Stop being stupid. You're going to ruin her life." He would end with, "I think you have rocks in your head."

In critical times like those, my father's words cut deep. As a union leader in Bayonne, New Jersey, he had to be a diplomat on many fronts and an astute listener. He had to uncover the hidden meanings behind what people said and their intentions. His life depended on it. His words resonate with me to this day. "Russ, people will tell you what you want to hear, okay? You have to listen to those words and find out what their true meaning is." My father's yellow hardhat had a black question mark in the center. As a child, this was way above my ability to conceptualize. However, as certain situations arose in my life, I would hear my father's words and just laugh to myself, thinking how spot-on the old man had been. His teaching made me think about those people we considered icons growing up. When the movie stars would come to town, my mother would get all excited, but my father would just say, "They're just people, but because they're on TV, I should kiss their ass?"

This was a constant in my home. Completely different thought processes from two people; many times, it was hilarious listening to them verbally spar. The back and forth was always at light speed. One day, our family was taking a walk down the boardwalk in Daytona Beach, taking in the sights, when the crowd of people ahead began moving quickly out of the way of three bikers strutting their colors. My father saw them coming straight at us, put his hand on my mother, and moved her to the left, and my sister and I followed. My father stood there looking straight at the bikers with laser focus. The bikers, when they caught sight of my father, separated and walked around him. My heart was racing, but then we resumed sightseeing and my father looked at me and said, "I'll be goddamned if I step out of the way of those assholes. They don't intimidate me!" As in every situation, my father was prepared for the worst-case scenario. He had always helped people, for as long I can remember, but he was also a warrior. He never started any trouble, never drank, and didn't smoke, but if someone drew first blood, it was on.

The nuns would tell me that I was going to burn in hell, as a form of discipline, and tell me that when I was on my deathbed, I would call out to God for forgiveness. Even as a kid, I was thinking, *Calling out for forgiveness!? What the fuck for? I didn't do anything!* As an adult, if I were on my deathbed, I would not call out for forgiveness. I would take a plane ride to 30,000 feet, jump out with no parachute, hit terminal velocity, fall through a ten-story glass building, land in a wood chipper that would spray my blood on a wall, saying, "Don't Pray for Me." Too extreme? I don't think so!

I tried to give you a visual of my death to remember those key words, like in a song. I understand now that if we are going to change medicine and go up against the titans of the industry, we have to educate people using visuals, music, and stories. Tell me your phone number and I would have to repeat it a few times or write it down to remember. But how many of us can still sing that song from the 80s, "867-5309"? Put it to music and it becomes unforgettable. Tell me a good joke one time, I'll remember it. Our brains are hardwired for stories, which is why every song has a hook. With my team, social media, and the Russ Scala YouTube channel, I need to find the hook that will resonate with people. I want them to learn from our content and share it. These ideas can change the world very quickly. I've developed high-level treatment protocols not offered at the Mayo Clinic. We have to develop videos and research to counteract all the leading medical institutions that will try to shoot us down. This content is far too complicated for regular folks to understand and apply to their lives, or to encourage them to take charge of their health without physicians who just write prescriptions that cause more damage. The content we need to develop for people has to be simple, like, "We are all biochemically unique." This basic truth allows us to get away from sweeping generalizations of treatments and customize programs based on every person's unique metabolism, lab work, and genetic profile.

Listening, creativity, and flow are three areas that allow my team to develop killer content that locks into a person's brain fast and encourages them to repeat and explain it to friends and family. If we can do this, we can change the world. I remember when I left the

SWAT team and started training and racing long-distance triathlons. If someone back in the late 80s or early 90s had said, "Russ, you're killing yourself," I never would have believed them. It is this fact—this stubbornness—that I have to keep front and center when considering how people will react and respond to our ideas.

One of my clients, who weighs 400 pounds, carries a special chair with him wherever he goes. He is a very smart man and has a certain outlook on life, which he shares. I also have clients who are recovering drug addicts. When my obese friend was making judgements about how weak he thought drug addicts were, he never considered that he was a carbohydrate addict. The fact is, you can do heroin, methadone, and other opiates for years and still be standing, but his obesity was going to kill him in a few years. Based on his lab work, he was already the victim of a heart attack; it just hadn't happened yet. His obesity is totally acceptable in society, but the heroin addict is seen as a criminal. Interesting, when you think about it. In my mind, I see addiction no differently than cancer or diabetes; again, we have to change the song in our head. Try telling a bodybuilder that he or she is killing him or herself. When these people look in the mirror, body dysmorphia takes over their minds and they see a small person, not a shredded Goliath that has been training for years. I've always immersed myself deeply into the culture of my clients, as this is the only way I can show them a way out. As I move away from designing advanced eleventh-hour interventions and move towards creating content, songs, movies, and books with my team, I'll still tap into my insatiable passion to effect change, but now I can do it on a scale that will reach millions of people!

Chapter Fourteen

DO THE VOODOO YOU DO

As I've aged, I've learned that I don't deal with trauma as well as I did when I was younger. Losing my folks without warning, the suddenness of it all, had me in a tailspin. I knew that the only way though this was to focus on my own biochemistry, particularly my prefrontal cortex. I had to eliminate all my bad thoughts, which is why running with a heart rate of 120 was so important for my recovery. What I did so well when helping other people, I now had to apply for myself. This brain hack needed to happen fast. I did bloodwork, consulted with my physicians, and adjusted my nootropics to keep my neurotransmitter levels elevated. The combination of lithium, testosterone, nicotine, GABA, and thyroid T3 was in my metabolic tool kit. Certain combinations, when calibrated, can cause extreme relaxation.

Of course, I also had to do my part, such as keeping a metabolic diary of what was working for me and discarding what wasn't. Writing this book was the beginning of my therapy; each chapter I wrote helped me relax. Good thoughts of my parents often came back when I focused on the specific details of our conversations. Those good times made me smile, and I realized how lucky I was to have them in my life as I passed from my twenties into my thirties… when life was kicking my ass. The words of my father resonated within me.

I often thought about the simple, uncaring words I would hear from supervisors while on the job: "When members of my crew are in a bad place, they had better man up and get over it." That should have been on a tee shirt. I've learned that everyone handles traumatic situations in different ways. For me, going through such an ordeal at this time in my life added more layers to my already thick skin.

After more than forty years in medicine, there's not a day that goes by when I don't think, *What can I do to just wake up this broken medical system? How can I impact the health of thousands of people?* When I was in graduate school, I got to data mine the best PhDs in business development, bounce ideas around, brainstorm, and talk about emerging medical markets. Remember, content is the new oil. I knew it would be a gold mine if my team could distill highly complex metabolic functions into a format that adults and children could understand and apply to their own behavior. *Game on,* I thought. Simple phrases that resonate and send a message like, "You're not what you eat, but what you absorb," speak to the new research on the microbiome, the flora in the intestinal tract. There are over a thousand different species of bacteria that live in our gut and help to keep us healthy. In fact, the first sip of breast milk that a mom gives her newborn goes right to the gut and starts growing that extremely beneficial flora to intensify immune surveillance. This thinking opens the door to talking about the gut/brain connection and why it's better to pull nutrients out of food, rather than just swallowing synthetic vitamins. On the cellular level, the body knows what's best for its intricate system, as multiple layers of complexity and the interconnection of multiple metabolic systems are needed to protect us. I knew that by using the internet, I could reach thousands of people. YouTube was a killer platform to easily educate people and give them that "Aha!" moment. Could I change people's thinking and transform knowledge into behavior with a three-minute video? The strategy was to give them a basic understanding of all the new research on disease prevention and performance as we age, and provide them with information that they would never hear from their physicians.

I'm always thinking, talking, and obsessing about the one keystone behavior that people will respond to. A keystone behavior is a behavior that, when started, is able to change other behaviors. A great example is weight loss. When done right, a person is happy, motivated, starts to exercise, buys new clothes, and surrounds themselves with a new community of like-minded folks. However, finding this behavior, as you can imagine, is difficult. I identify certain pathologies in people. I see athletes and I see worried healthy people who just want to feel better. Each group requires a different approach. I remember trying to get cops, firemen, and paramedics to back off the simple carbohydrates when my training partners shifted to the ketogenic diet in 1988, but because I lacked the behavior training skills back then, I just gave up. This group has the highest risk of heart disease out of any demographic, and now we know why. Carbohydrates cause the burst of the feel-good neurotransmitter, serotonin, and all the emergency service personnel were addicted. How else do you quiet your brain and get to sleep after handling a high-intensity emergency scene?

Twenty years later, my sleep is still disrupted. It's a constant battle to monitor my metabolism just to stay mentally healthy.

Many venture capitalists came to me with new ideas. I looked at new business startups like a living organism, ripping through hundreds of business case studies. I would ask, "Will this new business evolve to be successful or will it die and go bankrupt?" My studies in this area were not as fascinating as the performance enhancement research, but I was making it work after finishing my master's. I've come up with a few game changers, but whether or not I can pull the trigger with investors has yet to be seen. I know that social media is lighting the fuse for massive cultural change and the people will soon take charge of their health, rather than relying purely on their physicians.

I've always researched trends in medicine, such as who the movers and shakers are and who is simply looking for an ROI on another drug that only treats symptoms. An ideal example of what's happening is the drug Lovasa. It's an omega-3 fatty acid that you have to get from your physician. We all know the benefits of omega-3 fatty acids, but Big Pharma saw the opportunity to turn a nutrient into a revenue stream while also saving billions in testing and designing a new drug, when people can just take omega-3s on their own.

Seeing how select groups of people were using social media to educate, inform, and save lives gave me the necessary push to jump back in the game when my endurance and passion was at a critical low point. I've educated physicians for years and a few truly want to further their knowledge of nutritional medicine, diet, and hormonal replacement and practice beyond the standard of care, which is basically controlled by Big Pharma. I've sat with hundreds of cardiologists over the past twenty years and showed each of them my research about fat not causing heart attacks. Because of their training, many never believe this fact, so it's much easier to educate people who have no medical training.

Now I see people with no medical training who have successfully turned around their diabetes on their own by doing research, experimenting, gathering data, and sharing their knowledge with tens of thousands of people in their social media groups. As Big Pharma continues to advertise drugs on TV, there has been a massive shift in people canceling their cable TV and customizing their own channels of interest. If you think about it, people customize their homes, their cars, and their business, so if research shows that we are all biochemically unique, then customizing our health is the next logical step. Every person on the planet has different nutritional deficiencies and needs different dietary combinations of protein, fat, and carbohydrates. Many are now using technology and lab work to determine what that tailored mix is for them.

To develop an advanced treatment protocol, I must be face-to-face with clients and spend hours learning about their behavior, job, family, current medications, friends, and how they view their current situation. I need to hear, in their own words, what has brought them to this point in their lives. No one wakes up one day and decides to be an alcoholic or get hooked on heroin. It's a process, so treatment must be customized to each person.

In order for me to trigger my creative side, I have to be up at 4 a.m. This is the best time for me, a leftover ritual from being a paramedic. Responding to emergency calls required me to stay jacked in and hyperalert, which did not make for a healthy lifestyle. Now, while developing advanced treatment protocols, I have had to find flow and stop the constant parade of energy and excitement in my head. I can make magic happen, but getting my brain to its sweet spot is always a task. Since I've been on the ketogenic diet and fasting, I just wake up at 4 a.m., as though I'm flipping on a light switch. Back when I was racing, pounding down the carbohydrates, PowerBars, bagels, and pasta, it took 60 minutes for me to clear my head enough to get going. I was always in a fog. Finding my flow, where I start dropping screens in my mind to make connections, is a self-indulgent art form, almost like lucid dreaming. It takes practice, and to get here, I had to use a combination of nicotine, caffeine, lithium, cocoa, and maca. This started as a brain hack to change my behavior. However, as my skills and research evolved, so did I. I know my own body and make changes on the fly, so this advanced nootropic protocol is light years away from the masses just taking a handful of vitamins. The leading neurological research teams took me by the hand years ago. People wonder how we can develop advanced brain rehabilitation protocols. Well, think about it for a second. I've been researching brain injuries since the 1980s when my best friend and fellow firefighter committed suicide by shooting himself in the chest with a .357 Magnum. I had missed all the signs. Now, I don't miss things. I've done my research.

At 4 a.m., I would often drive to get coffee. There was something about the drive that was calming for me. There was no one on the road; it was surreal, and I liked that feeling. At that time, I own the night. I would arrive at the 7/11 and buy a small coffee; it didn't matter what kind. In that situation, the coffee was the delivery system for the nootropics. I would grab an extra empty cup and then mix the cocoa and maca powders with the coffee, pouring it from one cup to the other a few times. This was to make sure the mix was consistent, without any residue left at the bottom. I would get back in the car and sip the nootropic brew while driving back. Once I arrived home, I would take two 5-milligram tablets of lithium. Bipolar patients take 300 milligrams, just to give you some perspective on dosing. I would then grab a small cigar called a Padron, go out to the back porch with a pad and start writing. My best moments of flow have come from this ritual, but I've experimented for years and I like turning the metabolic radio dials, many hours of fine tuning, taking notes, paying attention to mood, sleep, energy levels, and lab work... oh and vomiting a few times along the way... it's hard to avoid that. Also, remember to go slow; test, don't guess. When writing protocols (and this book), I would start by making a circle on the page in the center. I would write the topic and then draw lines out from the center for the bullet points. I would focus on the foundation of the research. This level of creativity lasts for about two hours, but that's all I need. I can write a first draft in that time and send it to my research team or editor. My stream-of-consciousness writing is not for the faint of heart.

The venture capitalists that I've met have said, "Russ, you can't scale this... it will never be successful." These idiots never understood that I *loved* what I was doing. I didn't care about scaling a business. This shortsighted thinking is why medicine is broken. As a kid, my family doctor made house calls and knew our whole family. When I would meet with these venture capital guys, I would watch them eat, talk about money, and drink like fish. I would think, *These motherfuckers are going to die screaming.* I now see people getting answers and taking care of themselves and family members. This is a powerful movement that is taking place, and it is only going to continue.

Current events signal a paradigm shift in medicine. It's happening in real time, as Dr. Eric Topol emphasized in his book, *The Patient Will See You Now*, which is a *New York Times* best seller. Dr. Topol served as chairman of cardiovascular medicine at the Cleveland Clinic and is currently the founder and director of Scripps Translational Science Institute in La Jolla, California. He was one of the first researchers that questioned the safety of the cholesterol drug, Vioxx, which was eventually pulled from the market.

There is a serious shift in thinking going on. People are sick and tired of Big Pharma just throwing an endless stream of drugs at them.

They want to (and will) improve their quality of life without the crutch of a physician. It's happening all over social media. People are monitoring their sleep patterns, diet, blood glucose, and ketones with advanced, inexpensive technologies. People are doing their own lab work and then corroborating the results with online resources that can guide them to wellness without multiple medications that simply treat symptoms, and not the cause.

I find it truly exciting to watch the passion and dedication of regular people who have more knowledge than 99.9% of physicians. I do believe that regular people will change medicine forever. Movies based on true stories, like *Lorenzo's Oil,* starring Susan Sarandon, and *First Do No Harm*, starring Meryl Streep, show how this can and does happen.

Think about this for a second... what do diabetes, heart disease, cancer, obesity and dementia all have in common? The answer is insulin. That's right... insulin. Now, this might blow your hair back. If you incorporate the ketogenic diet and intermittent fasting, you will impact more metabolic pathways than any drug that is currently on the market, since conventional medicine compartmentalizes these diseases with separate treatments and separate drugs for each condition. People are now understanding the science and not buying into the slick marketing of medicine as a business. *"First, do no harm..."* my ass!

Here's a key lesson, folks. I don't want to put you to sleep with scientific research, but here we go. On the cellular level, when the mitochondria create energy (ATP), carbohydrates are not needed. Now, just by knowing this, you will be far ahead of any college professor or physician, as well as any nutritional expert, because they are all teaching science that's simply not true. While I'm ranting, let's go here for a minute. Fat loss is not about calories or exercise. I'll show people a vial of insulin or a pill vial with the medication prednisone inside and ask, "How many calories does this medication have?" I tell them that insulin and prednisone have zero calories, but isn't it interesting that if you take these meds, you will gain fat? Fat loss or gain is hormonally regulated. Again, it's not about calories and exercise.

People are going on the ketogenic diet and combining intermittent fasting to reverse diabetes. I've seen this happen hundreds of times. The lab work doesn't lie. Dr. Jason Fung is on the tip of the spear educating people. His book, *The Obesity Code*, just plunged a dagger into the heart of conventional diabetes treatment. This is one man, and there are many more people across the US on Facebook telling their stories and sharing information. This creates questions where everyone can learn exponentially. Now, they will make mistakes, of course, but what they're doing on social media is not being done in physicians' offices. That's powerful. Talk about the tipping point! And here it is...

Imagine that your physician wants to write a prescription for an ADHD drug for your child or put your aging parents on a statin. We know these drugs cause damage on the cellular level. You can take control of your family's health and say no. As I mentioned before, I can't stop thinking about taking people from their homes into assisted living centers in their sixties. Years later, as I worked in the anti-aging nutritional and hormonal replacement market, I saw people of the same age having a ball, laughing, exercising, taking trips, and riding their bikes around Europe. This is why I do what I do. It's my mission to improve the quality of life for people. I have no kids, no wife, and I don't watch sports... I've always felt like a warrior on the front lines of this crucial battle. Maybe that's why I felt totally at peace on emergency scenes. I felt like helping people is what I've been put here to do. Now, don't get me wrong, I also have a passion for educating a team around me composed of select physicians, researchers, and wicked-smart people that give a shit at the end of the day. When you look into someone's eyes, within seconds, you can tell if they care. After what I've recently been through, I have no expectations from people. Zero. Zilch. Fortunately, by writing the lines in this book, I feel better than when I started. If anything in this book resonates with people, that's great, but if not, I still accomplished my mission.

When I think about the thousands of medical offices across the US where tens of thousands of people wait every day, only to receive prescriptions that are damaging their metabolism, the task seems overwhelming. However, the social media model of education gives me hope that my efforts to change medicine are not in vain. I trust that at least one person I educate will share what they learn with friends and family. This viral sharing of real science will gradually shift the thinking of conventional medicine. We'll soon be using nutrition as part of the cellular healing process, whether the application is heart disease, dementia, or performance enhancement. Ground zero is correcting nutritional deficiencies with functional foods and understanding that your metabolism is unique from anyone else's.

Everybody and every body… has a story.

GET IN TOUCH WITH RUSS

Scala Precision Health
www.ScalaPrecisionHealth.com

Institute of Nutritional Medicine & Cardiovascular Research
www.PersonalizedHealthInstitute.com

Facebook: www.facebook.com/russ.scala
YouTube: www.youtube.com/user/RussScala

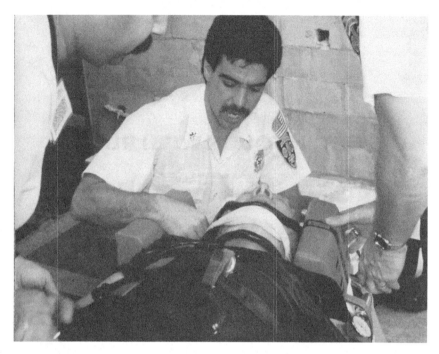

Responding to emergency calls—I loved it, but it took a toll on my health. Collateral damage.

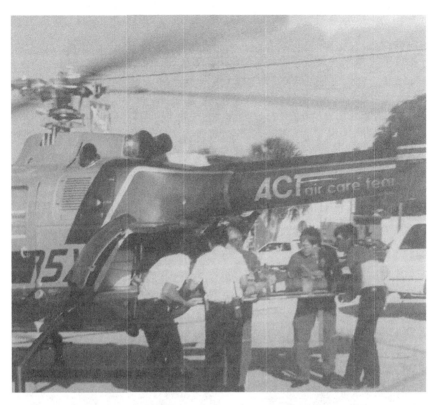

The first time we air-vacked a patient to the new trauma
center at Orlando Regional Medical Center.

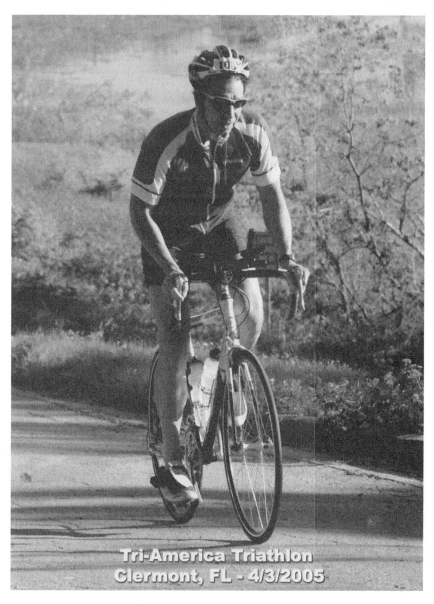

Tri-America Triathlon
Clermont, FL - 4/3/2005

I didn't realize it at the time, but I really damaged my
metabolism with training and racing.

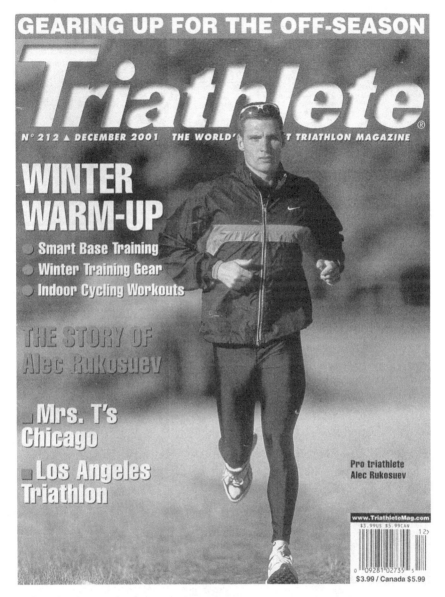

Alec Rukosuev was the first pro athlete we tested in 1996.

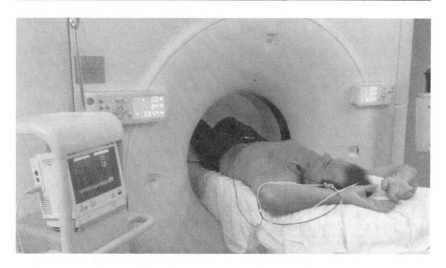

We discovered why extremely fit athletes were having heart attacks, which scared me… so I got into a CAT scan myself!

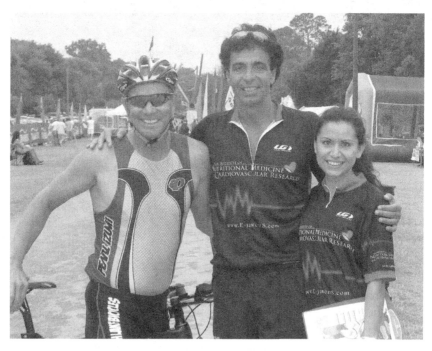

Harry Nichols, my good buddy, is no longer with us. He died of a heart attack at age 42. He was one of the fittest guys I knew.

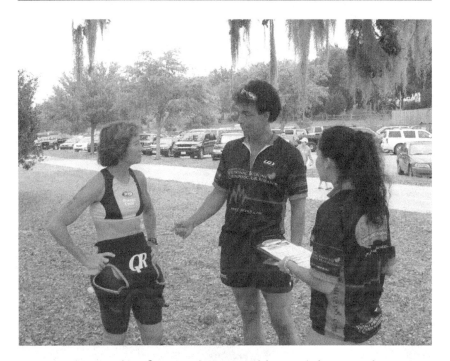

Gathering data from endurance athletes while researching
cardiac arrhythmias.

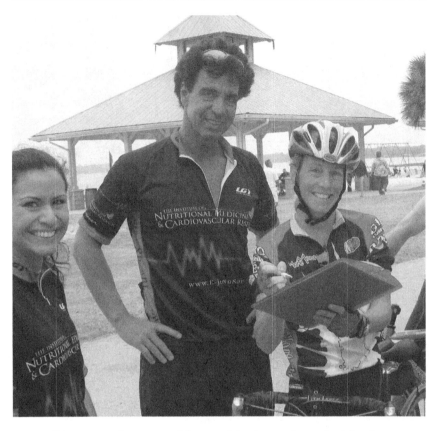

Testing endurance athletes with elevated cortisol levels.

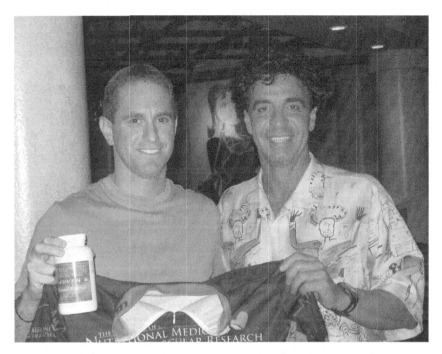

My buddy, Scott Levitt, was the first endurance athlete client who'd had a heart attack for whom we created a protocol.

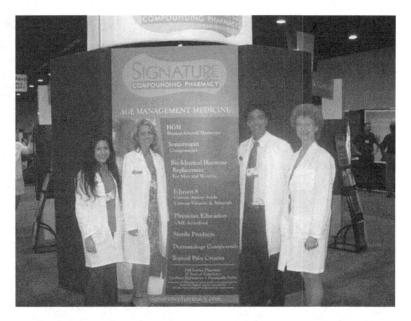

Las Vegas 2005: Presenting our research and new
formulations to the anti-aging medical community.

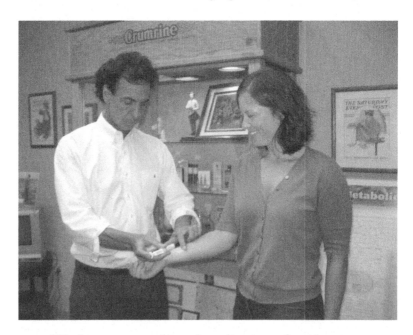

Working on transdermal application of medication.

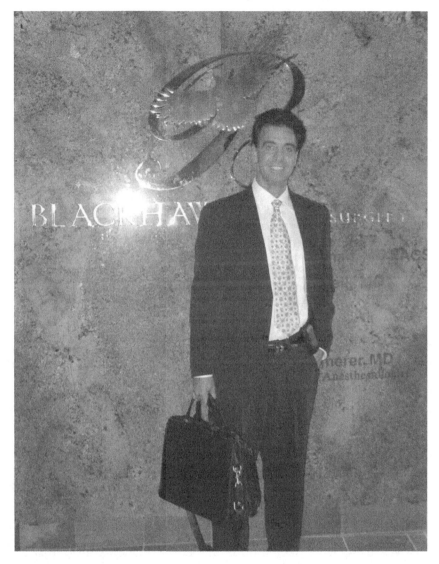

Office of the first plastic surgeon I trained in hormonal
replacement therapy in 2006.

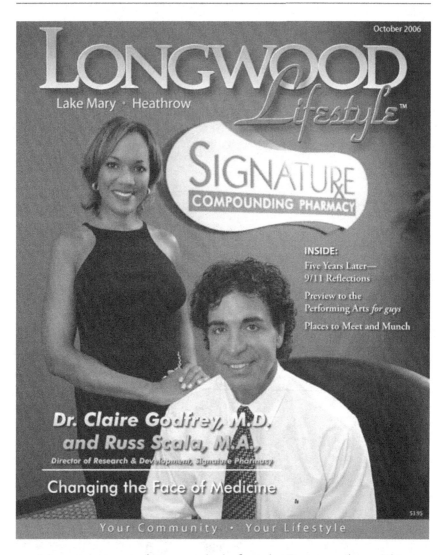

Magazine cover taken months before the Signature bust. This picture got shot around the national news for two months.

The New York Times

≡   Q

4 Tied to Pharmacy Are Arrested in Inquiry Into Steroid Sales

By NICHOLAS CONFESSORE
FEBRUARY 28, 2007

ALBANY, Feb. 27 — Federal and state investigators on Tuesday arrested four people with ties to a pharmacy in Orlando, Fla., that law enforcement officials said accounted for a large part of the national market in steroids and other performance enhancers that are sold illegally online.

The arrests followed a two-year investigation by the Albany County district attorney into Internet drug sales in New York State. The investigation spanned at least three states, and included numerous people reported to be customers of the pharmacy, including current and former Major League Baseball players, National Football League players, college athletes, coaches and doctors.

At least two dozen other individuals are expected to face indictment in New York, according to P. David Soares, the district attorney for Albany County, including several doctors and pharmacists. At a news conference in Orlando on Tuesday, he

New York Times coverage of the Signature bust.

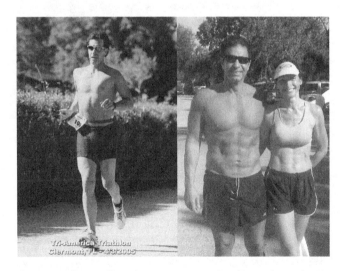

Before & after: After damaging my body with endurance training, it took four years to repair myself, using nutritional support and hormonal replacement.

THE INSTITUTE OF

NUTRITIONAL MEDICINE
&CARDIOVASCULAR RESEARCH

" The e-Juven 8 program, through testing, uncovered specific nutritional deficiencies related to my own unique metabolism. I'm a cancer survivor training to ride across the U.S. with Lance Armstrong in the tour of Hope. It was critical for my training and immunity that I get a program that is customized for me and only me. I recommend this program to anyone who wants to see what is really going on inside our bodies. "

Wendy Chioji
News Anchor
and Cancer Survivor

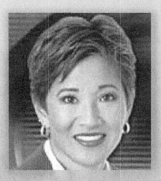

Testimonial after creating a program for local celebrity Wendy Chioji.

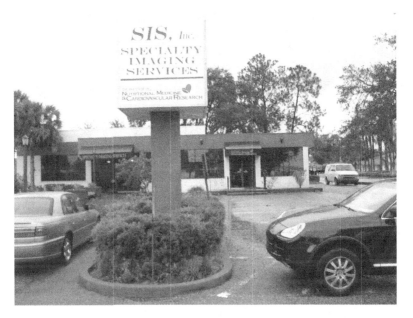

The Institute's first location, where we used advanced
imaging to track muscle wasting.

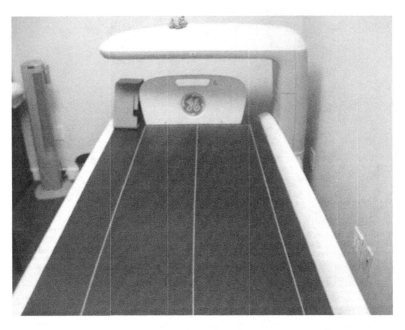

The iDexa machine that measures body-to-muscle ratios.

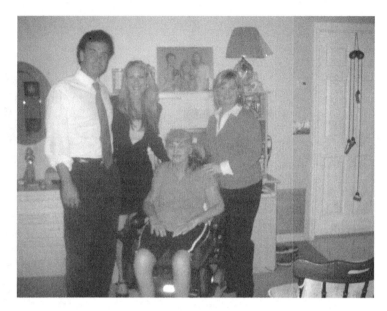

Our first eleventh-hour intervention. This woman had
90 days to live.

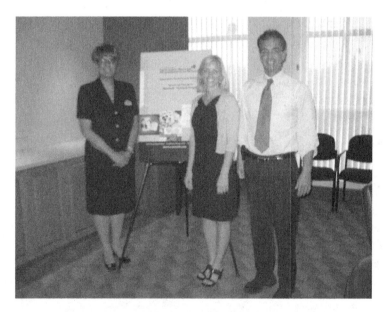

Former Bethune-Cookman College president Trudie Reed
going over her test results.

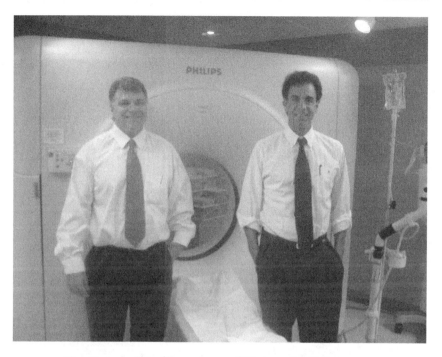

Dr. George Stanley, owner of University Diagnostic
Institute, was always a phone call away while I was
formulating my brain rehabilitation program.

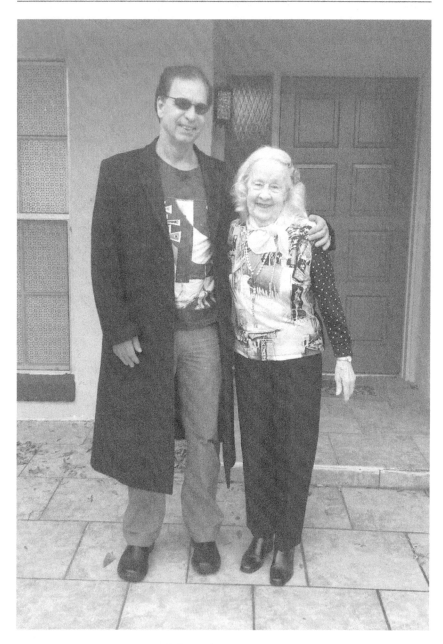

Me and my mom.

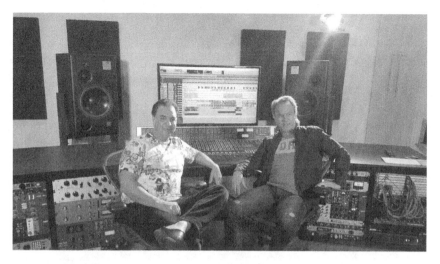

With Erick Pace in the godAmsterdams' recording studio.

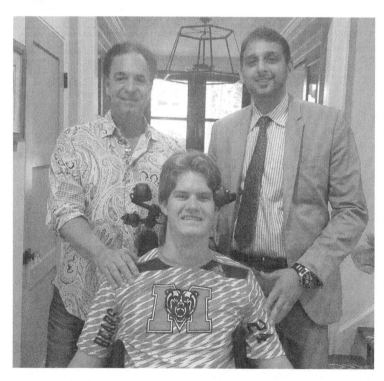

John Michael Night, paralyzed by a stroke, has required our
most advanced protocol to date.

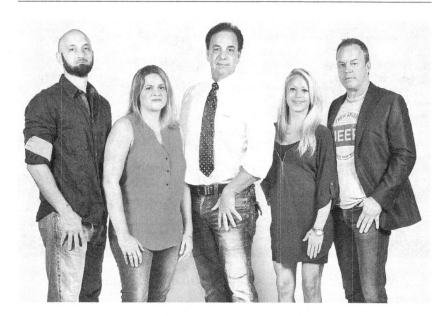

The Team: Trent Duncan, Chrissy Mifsud, Russ Scala,
Michelle Conti, Erick Pace

Photo by Jacque Brund

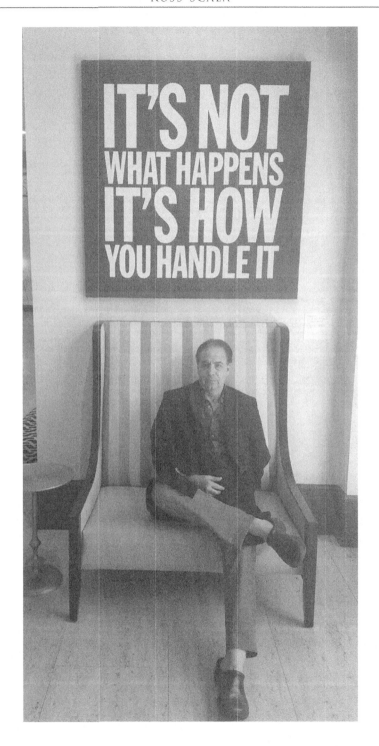